THE
Green
Tea
Book

AVERY

a member of

Penguin Group (USA) Inc.

New York

THE
Green
Tea
Book

The Science-Backed
"Miracle Cure"

Lester A. Mitscher, Ph.D., *and*

Victoria Dolby Toews, MPH

AVERY

Published by the Penguin Group

Penguin Group (USA) Inc., 375 Hudson Street, New York, New York 10014, USA •
Penguin Group (Canada), 90 Eglinton Avenue East, Suite 700, Toronto, Ontario M4P 2Y3,
Canada (a division of Pearson Penguin Canada Inc.) • Penguin Books Ltd, 80 Strand, London
WC2R 0RL, England • Penguin Ireland, 25 St Stephen's Green, Dublin 2, Ireland (a division of
Penguin Books Ltd) • Penguin Group (Australia), 250 Camberwell Road, Camberwell, Victoria 3124,
Australia (a division of Pearson Australia Group Pty Ltd) • Penguin Books India Pvt Ltd,
11 Community Centre, Panchsheel Park, New Delhi–110 017, India • Penguin Group (NZ),
67 Apollo Drive, Rosedale, North Shore 0632, New Zealand (a division of Pearson
New Zealand Ltd) • Penguin Books (South Africa) (Pty) Ltd, 24 Sturdee Avenue,
Rosebank, Johannesburg 2196, South Africa

Penguin Books Ltd, Registered Offices: 80 Strand, London WC2R 0RL, England

Most Avery books are available at special quantity discounts for bulk purchase for sales promotions, premiums, fund-raising, and educational needs. Special books or book excerpts also can be created to fit specific needs. For details, write Penguin Group (USA) Inc. Special Markets, 375 Hudson Street, New York, NY 10014.

Library of Congress Cataloging-in-Publication Data

Mitscher, Lester A.
The green tea book : the science-backed "miracle cure" / Lester A. Mitscher, Victoria Dolby Toews.
p.   cm.
Includes bibliographical references and index.
ISBN 978-1-58333-302-0
1. Green tea—Therapeutic use. 2. Green tea—Health aspects. I. Dolby Toews, Victoria. II. Title.
RM251.M563   2008   2007032840
615'.321—dc22

Printed in the United States of America
1 3 5 7 9 10 8 6 4 2

BOOK DESIGN BY NICOLE LAROCHE

Neither the publisher nor the authors are engaged in rendering professional advice or services to the individual reader. The ideas, procedures, and suggestions in this book are not intended as a substitute for consulting with a physician. All matters regarding health require medical supervision. Neither the authors nor the publisher shall be liable or responsible for any loss or damage allegedly arising from any information or suggestion in this book.

While the authors have made every effort to provide accurate telephone numbers and Internet addresses at the time of publication, neither the publisher nor the authors assume any responsibility for errors, or for changes that occur after publication. Further, the publisher does not have any control over and does not assume any responsibility for author or third-party websites or their content.

To Betty, together always
—LAM

Just to Elizabeth (she knows why)
—VDT

Contents

Thank God for tea! What would the world do without tea? How did it exist? I am glad I was not born before tea.

—Letter from Sidney Smith (1771–1845)

Green Tea and Its Health Benefits

Since ancient times, green tea has been prized as a traditional tonic for keeping the body and soul in good condition. In modern times, scientific studies have confirmed many of the traditionally held beliefs about green tea. It seems that every few months another scientific study confirms the healthful potential of green tea that was first recorded by a Chinese emperor more than 4,000 years ago.

When the first edition of this book was originally published, almost a decade ago, our readers must have been motivated about green tea, because back then you had to work a bit to purchase green tea if you were outside of Asia. You probably had to travel to a specialty tea store or a health food store. Today, the rest of the world is learning what we've known all along: Green tea is great for you! Today, green tea (and even oolong tea and white tea) is readily found in the average supermarket, and even as ready-to-drink beverages at corner convenience stores. And hand-in-hand with this increased availability comes the financial growth of the tea industry. Over the past fifteen years, tea sales have more than tripled to the greater than $6 billion industry it is today.

Some of the most exciting research involves the link between green tea and the prevention of cancer. Additionally, green tea eases the adverse effects of cancer therapies, such as radiation and chemotherapy. Other research shows that tea, and green tea in particular, bolsters the heart's resistance to cardiovascular diseases, prevents dental cavities, lengthens a tea drinker's life span, detoxifies the body, aids in weight loss, decreases cholesterol levels, protects skin from sun damage, relieves mental distress, and boosts the immune function. And over the years, the research in these areas has gotten more positive.

Just Three Cups a Day . . .

The magic number for tea seems to be the very pleasant and manageable three to six cups per day. Numerous studies keep coming back to this number time and again. Here are some additional statistics:

- Drinking any amount of tea regularly makes it 40 percent more likely that a person who has a heart attack will survive and still be alive three years later.
- One to two cups daily lowers the risk of severe hardening of the arteries (atherosclerosis) by 46 percent.
- Two cups a day leads to a 50 percent reduction in heart disease in general.
- Three cups daily slashes the risk of having a heart attack by 43 percent.
- Three cups a day lowers LDL ("bad") cholesterol levels.
- Four cups a day greatly lowers the risk of skin cancer.
- Five cups daily lowers stroke risk by 62 percent in women and 42 percent in men.
- Five cups a day reduces the chances of developing breast cancer. (The bullet points above all refer to studies that will be discussed in more depth later in the book.)

A note about cup sizes: When people around the world pour themselves a "cup of tea" they might be talking about very different cup sizes. In Japan, the average cup size for tea is a petite 3.5 ounces. In Europe, teacups tend to hold about 5 ounces, while in the United States, a mug of tea contains a weighty 8 ounces. Throughout this book, a cup of tea refers to the 1-cup measurement, equivalent to 8 ounces (237 milliliters).

Scientists working around the world have identified the substanc green tea that provide the majority of its health benefits. These "magic bullets" of health protection primarily are a class of chemicals called polyphenols, which we'll discuss in more detail later. It is interesting to note that many studies documenting the health benefits of tea have been conducted in countries where black tea is the typical drink. Although black tea does contain some polyphenols, green tea's polyphenol levels are far higher. If black tea has already impressed scientists, imagine how much greater the health protection of green tea is believed to be. You don't have to make a leap of faith from "if the small amounts of polyphenols in black tea are good" to "the larger amounts in green tea will be even better," because research has already proven that green tea offers an astonishing array of life-enhancing and even life-preserving properties.

The "Secret Ingredients" of Tea

When modern researchers finally studied green tea, they confirmed what the Chinese had said for centuries: that green tea holds within it a special health-preserving and revitalizing power. For many years, however, most Western scientists had not been interested in hearing about the preventive and medicinal power of any herbs, let alone green tea. All this changed after research began to roll in showing that certain plants do indeed contain powerful health-promoting and even healing substances. This category of substances is known to researchers as phytonutrients.

Perhaps you've already heard about phytonutrients, or know them by another name, such as nutriceuticals, phytochemicals, phytomedicines, or functional food factors. Regardless of their label, they're all the same thing: naturally occurring compounds found in plants (*phyto* is the Greek word for "plant") that protect against disease and promote good health.

Plants use these compounds for their own survival. Many act in the plant as hormones, enzymes, pigments, or growth regulators. Others provide color, odor, and taste. Without phytonutrients, plants would not be able to protect themselves from free radicals, parasites, bacteria, viruses, insects, and injuries. Lucky for us, many of these benefits are transferred when we consume the plant or plant extract. Although phytonutrients are not nutrients in the traditional sense—that is, they don't provide energy or elements essential to the metabolic process—they have just as much effect on health as any vitamin or mineral.

By the 1950s, scientists thought that they had discovered all of the important elements in food. They were wrong. Only today are phyto-nutrients gaining the recognition they deserve. Even though researchers are actively investigating phytonutrients, some authorities estimate that 99 percent of phytonutrients have yet to be discovered! Fortunately, the phytonutrients in green tea are among those already documented as potent healers.

Because phytonutrients are a formidably large category, scientists divide them into several smaller classes to make them easier to understand. One of these classes is the polyphenols. Polyphenols are present in tea, and in apples, onions, red wine, and many other foods as well. Polyphenols are best known for being effective antioxidants, and the polyphenols in green tea are no exception. Throughout this book, you'll learn about the many ways in which the antioxidant effects of green tea's polyphenols counter-act free radicals and the diseases they would otherwise cause.

And now let's correct a misconception about tea. Many people think that caffeine-containing drinks, including tea, act as a diuretic and could potentially lead to dehydration instead of quenching your body's fluid needs. The origin of this line of thinking comes from studies that have people consume very large amounts of caffeine—equivalent to drinking eight cups of tea in one sitting. This amount of caffeine does in fact have a diuretic effect, promoting dehydration. But who would realistically drink this enormous amount of tea in one go? In real-world settings, drinking several cups of tea spread throughout the day does *not* have a diuretic effect, and the opposite is true—drinking tea keeps the body hydrated.[1] Incidentally, when brewed in the usual manner, the average cup of tea contains about half (50 milligrams) of the caffeine contained in the aver-age cup of coffee (100 milligrams).

Cultivation of Tea

The tea plant, technically known as *Camellia sinensis*, is cultivated in more than thirty different countries, most notably in China, Japan, India, and Sri Lanka (formerly known as Ceylon). Approximately 3.1 million tons of dried tea are produced each year. Of this, about 20 percent is green tea, less than 2 percent is oolong tea and white tea, and the balance of 78 percent is black tea.

Although green tea, black tea, white tea, and oolong tea are all derived from the single plant species *Camellia sinensis,* there are two major varieties of the tea plant: *sinensis* and *assamica.* The varieties are distinguished on the basis of leaf size. The *sinensis* variety has leaves five to twelve centimeters long, while the leaves of the *assamica* variety may measure up to twenty centimeters in length.

Tea is a hardy plant that grows best at higher altitudes with plenty of warm, rainy weather. Most commonly, tea plantations—or tea gardens as they are often called—are located in mountainous areas or near tropical jungles. Tea plants prosper in areas with foggy mornings, balmy days with temperatures of 65°F, and heavy yearly rainfalls. Most teas are grown in sedimentary soils that are slightly acidic. Much like wine, teas are identified by the area in which they were grown; and again like wine, each area is renowned for teas that have distinct flavor and character.

If they are left untended, tea bushes will continue growing to as much as forty feet in height, and certain impressive specimens have reached heights twice that, but bushes are generally cut back every few years for the convenience of the harvesters. Tended tea bushes will produce tea for up to fifty years, and some tea plants are reputed to be centuries old. After three years of growth, a tea bush is ready for its first harvest. To ensure the quality of the final product, tea plants are chosen for harvesting on the basis of "pubescence," indicated by hair growth on the underside of the leaves, and for an attractive green color.

Some tea is mechanically harvested, but the majority of tea crops are harvested by hand, much as they were hundreds of years ago in the tea gardens of Chinese emperors. Most of the harvesters are women, who walk between the rows of tea bushes plucking the leaves by hand and tossing them into baskets strapped to their backs. Hand harvesting remains superior to mechanical harvesting because for the highest-quality tea, care must be taken to pluck only the "flush" of the tea plant—the tender new growth on the pruned bush, consisting of two leaves and a bud. The tradition of plucking only the bud and two leaves to produce high-quality tea may affect more than just the tea's taste. Compared with the older leaves, this part of the tea plant is almost three times richer in polyphenols.[2]

Green tea and white tea undergo the simplest processing of all the teas, since the traditional goal is to preserve the fresh flavor of the tea, and an additional modern goal is to retain as much of the fresh leaf's chemical constituents as possible. After the fresh leaves have been plucked, the next step is to inactivate enzymes that would otherwise degrade the tea; this is accomplished either by steaming the leaves or pan firing them. This step is also included in the processing of black and oolong tea, but after a varying lapse of time. Next, the tea leaves are rolled to squeeze the juices to the surface of the leaf, and then they are dried in high-temperature air to reduce their moisture content. Black and oolong teas are allowed to undergo enzymatic oxidation, which helps develop their characteristic odor and flavor and alters their polyphenol content. The processed leaves are sifted through progressively smaller mesh sieves to sort them by size. The best teas are chosen from the largest leaves, and lower grades of tea continue down in size. The tea "dust" that is left is used for tea in tea bags. The final result is packaged and shipped around the world for millions of people to enjoy every day.

Varieties of Tea

There are many teas, but just one plant; all teas are produced from *Camellia sinensis,* and slight differences in processing methods result in the tea varieties. The four common tea types are green tea, black tea, oolong tea, and white tea. Note that "red tea," which is gaining in popularity in recent years, is not actually tea, since it doesn't come from the *Camellia sinensis* plant. (See "What's in Your Cup" on page 8.) Even so, red tea—also known as rooibos or red bush tea—does convey antioxidants and seems to prevent cancer. The Swedish botanist Linnaeus (originator of the two-part Latin names for plants) believed that there were two species of tea, the *viridis* (green tea) and the *bohea* (black tea). However, Robert Fortune, an English adventurer who masqueraded as a Chinese merchant in order to learn how to cultivate tea, discovered that green and black teas are, in fact, derived from the same plant.

Green Tea

Green tea is the palest in color, generally a subtle shade of light green or yellow. The green color comes primarily from chlorophyll extracted from the green leaves by hot water. After the tea leaves are picked, they are lightly processed to prevent some natural changes from taking place. Of greatest interest to this narrative is the auto-oxidation catalyzed by natural enzymes present in the freshly plucked leaves. If allowed to proceed unchecked, this oxidation would convert the tea progressively to oolong and then black tea. Light steaming or gentle heat, however, prevents this oxidation, thereby preserving important natural antioxidants in the leaves. The result is green tea. The auto-oxidation was originally thought to be caused by microbes and was called fermentation. This is now known not to be the case.

Black Tea

Black tea has a stronger flavor and darker color than green tea. These tea leaves have undergone considerable processing, including auto-oxidation, which produces the dark brown and even reddish color of "black" tea. Unfortunately, this process also chemically alters the polyphenols originally present in the tea, decreasing their antioxidant power. Despite its diminished health value, black tea is the most popular tea worldwide, constituting nearly 80 percent of all tea produced and drunk.

Oolong Tea

Oolong is Chinese for "black dragon," but despite its assertive name, oolong tea takes the middle road between green and black tea in all ways. The method used for processing oolong is the newcomer among tea-processing methods; it wasn't developed until the mid-nineteenth century. Oolong tea is partially auto-oxidized, so it is slightly stronger in taste than green tea but more delicate than the fully auto-oxidized black tea. The partial auto-oxidation process, though, means that oolong tea contains lower levels of polyphenols. Oolong tea is the least widely used; less than 2 percent of the yearly tea consumption is based on this variety.

White Tea

White tea is made from the youngest tea leaves and buds, which are lightly steamed and then dried. White tea, like green tea, contains very

What's in Your Cup?

Just because something is brewing in a tea cup, doesn't mean that it's actually tea. There are many warm drinks that get called "tea" in common parlance, but few of these drinks actually contain leaves from the *Camellia sinensis* plant. These so-called teas are more correctly referred to as *tisanes* (or herbal infusions). Tisanes are made from various herbs (leaves, stems, fruits, bark, flowers, and roots of plants) steeped in hot water; many are caffeine free.

Although there are hundreds, if not thousands, of herbs that could theoretically be used, a much smaller number generally make it into the teapot. These herbal tisanes are the ones that have a palatable (and in many cases very tasty!) flavor as well as many of them having stood the test of time—and modern scientific scrutiny—as effective herbal healers. It's been known since ancient times that herbal tisanes can be healing tonics to restore health to the body, mind, and spirit. Often several herbs with complementary effects are blended together in a tisane, with the addition of non-medicinal ingredients, such as cinnamon, cloves, orange peel, or even essential oils, for better flavor.

The following are some of the more popular tisanes:

Chamomile: Relaxes the body and is a digestive aid.
Echinacea: Supports the immune system to prevent or alleviate cold or flu symptoms.
Elderberry: Fights the flu.
Fennel: Aids digestion.
Ginger: Settles the stomach and quells motion sickness and morning sickness.
Ginseng: Stimulates the mind and body.
Maté (or yerbamate): Stimulates the body (due to caffeine content). Brewed from toasted wild holly leaves. Originates from Argentina, Brazil, and Paraguay.
Milk thistle: Supports liver health.
Nettle: Helps ease hay fever.

Peppermint: Aids digestion.

Red clover: Detoxifies the body and supports the body during menopause.

Red tea or Rooibos: Provides antioxidant and cancer-preventive properties. Made from needle-like leaves of a South African shrub. Similar in taste to black tea.

St. John's wort: Boosts mood.

Valerian: Promotes a sense of calm; sedative effects.

White willow: Eases pain.

little caffeine and very high levels of antioxidants. In fact, antioxidant levels in white tea are even slightly higher than those in green tea. Once brewed, white tea is very pale in color.

Tea: Traditional and Convenient Forms

Tea has always been a versatile drink—coming in several varieties and equally tasty hot as well as cold, and more than appropriate at any time of day or night. And tea won't put a dent in your pocketbook; tea made at home can cost as little as three cents a cup.

While brewing tea leaves loose in hot water is a satisfying way to make this beverage, when the tea bag was introduced back in 1904, the simple convenience of this handy packaging (and freedom from straining tea leaves) became an attractive option that increased tea's popularity. Today, as yet another move toward ease and convenience, tea is becoming increasingly available in ready-to-drink bottles that offer the utmost in expediency. For example, even mainstream soft drink companies are adding ready-to-drink green tea products to their lines. For those who like the taste and convenience, this is another alternative. However, making and drinking your own green tea will give the same effect and provide quite a relief to your wallet.

Many substances found in nature or made by scientists can prevent or treat the diseases that afflict mankind, yet each seems to have a drawback:

Some work for only one condition, for example, and others are expensive, inconvenient, or unpleasant. Green tea stands out because it is different from those substances. Not only does it boost immune function and help prevent cancer, heart disease, diabetes, and dental cavities, but it is easy to use, inexpensive, and tastes great! Clearly, there are many reasons to become a green tea consumer.

Health professionals caution that green tea does not cure disease. Rather it is viewed as a pleasant adjunct to exercise and a balanced diet. When used in conjunction with avoidance of high-risk behaviors it helps delay the onset and decrease the severity of disease and the inevitable decline of aging.

chapter one

A Medicine Chest of Good Health

Few herbs have as long or impressive a history as green tea. From time immemorial, tea has been thought to possess healing potential, and scientists today confirm that those beliefs do indeed hold merit. The first recorded use of green tea dates back more than 4,000 years, and even then, tea enthusiasts believed that this tasty drink could ward off disease and improve health. Since that early reference to green tea as a health elixir, an impressive amount of evidence has accumulated to link green tea with good health. From protecting the heart against any number of cardiovascular diseases to keeping teeth strong and healthy, green tea seems to do it all. Let's take a quick overview of the types of health protection afforded by green tea. (See, "Just Three Cups a Day . . ." on page 2 for a summary.) Later chapters will examine all of these benefits in more detail.

Investigating Traditional Health Claims for Tea

Tea, whether green, black, white, or oolong, has an impressive history as a healthful beverage. The famous Chinese tea master Lu Yu wrote in A.D. 780 that tea could cure headaches, body aches and pains, constipation, and depression. Over the centuries, many others have praised the healing properties of tea, and drinking green tea was even purported to have brought a thirteenth century Japanese official back from his death bed. Following are some of the other traditional health claims for tea:

- increases blood flow throughout the body
- stimulates mental clarity
- detoxifies the body
- boosts immunity
- preserves young-looking skin
- brightens the eyes
- aids digestion
- banishes fatigue
- prolongs the life span

For many years, scientists were skeptical about the health claims made by tea proponents. This skepticism was soon transformed into appreciation when researchers began scientific investigations into the disease-preventing properties of green tea and confirmed most of the health claims.

Green Tea and Cardiovascular Disease

One of the most impressive discoveries has been the effect that green tea has in bolstering the heart's resistance to cardiovascular diseases. Study after study has shown that drinking plenty of tea and consuming other foods rich in particular polyphenols (the main active ingredients in tea) reduces the risk of having a heart attack, and decreases the likelihood of dying from a heart attack if one does occur. In fact, drinking just three cups a day slashes your risk of having a heart attack by 43 percent. Tea drinking also protects the blood vessels that feed the heart and brain; men who have the highest intakes of polyphenols from tea and other foods have 42 percent fewer strokes than men with low intakes.

Green tea guards against cardiovascular diseases in a number of ways. Specifically, drinking green tea lowers total cholesterol levels and results in a better cholesterol profile (that is, the ratio of LDL-cholesterol to HDL-cholesterol is improved). Research shows that the cholesterol levels of men who drink nine or more cups of green tea daily are lower than those of men who drink two or fewer cups.[1] When animals are fed a diet that raises their cholesterol levels, the addition of extract prevents the expected increase in cholesterol levels.[2] In green tea extract may be just as effective as aspirin for reducing platelet aggregation, or "thinning the blood."[3] Blood pressure is also lower in tea drinkers.[4]

Green Tea and Cancer

Green tea's indisputable antioxidant activity led cancer researchers to investigate the possibility that green tea might protect a person against developing cancer. Animal studies have indicated that green tea extract protects against both the initiation and promotion stages of cancer. "The inhibitory activity is believed to be mainly due to the antioxidative properties and possible antiproliferative effects of polyphenolic compounds in green and black tea," said researchers in the *Journal of the National Cancer Institute.* Specifically, in animal studies green tea extract has been shown to prevent cancers of the lung, breast, prostate, liver, skin, esophagus, and colon.[5]

Recently, researchers at Purdue University proposed that a cell surface protein (called t-NOX) is involved in the loss of control of regulated cell growth that is characteristic of many cancers. Certain compounds, including green tea catechins, interact with this rogue protein, disabling it with the result that tumor cells fail to thrive. This would appear to be another mechanism whereby green tea inhibits cancer cells.[6]

An enzyme system in the liver, called P450, can contribute to cancer by producing carcinogens from certain ingested or inhaled substances. Once again, as protective agents, green tea's polyphenols come through with flying colors. The antioxidative properties of green tea extract have been shown to inhibit P450 as a potential source of cancer-causing agents. Not all of the research on tea has shown cancer protection. The results of some earlier studies have been inconsistent, with some indicating benefits while others showed no benefit or even an increased risk of cancer associated with drinking tea. In order to get to the bottom of this equivocal evidence, researchers from the University of Minnesota School of Public Health correlated the tea drinking habits of 35,369 women and their incidence of cancer over an eight-year period. The women who drank green or black tea regularly showed a lower risk of developing cancers of the upper digestive tract, colon, and rectum. Urinary tract cancer was also less common in the tea drinkers. Women who frequently drank tea lowered their cancer risk by one-third, compared with those who rarely or never drank tea. Overall, drinking two or more cups of tea daily reduced the risk of cancer by 10 percent.[7] Some of the reports of increased cancer risk associated with tea-drinking have been traced to the combined effects of a poor diet and the habit of drinking tea at scaldingly hot temperatures.

Green Tea and Longevity

The key to living a longer life may be another secret brewing in green tea. Researchers investigated this possibility by following the lives of 3,380 Japanese women for nine years. Because these women were practitioners of chanoyu (the Japanese tea ceremony), they were presumed to be greater-than-average green tea drinkers. Compared with the mortality rates of other Japanese women during the period of the study, fewer of the green tea drinkers died, "indicating the possibility that green tea is a protective factor" against premature death.[8]

The overall health-promoting effect of polyphenols may account for green tea's role in longevity. Green tea has a stimulating effect on the immune system because its polyphenols boost production of immune system cells. Researchers hypothesize that this stimulation of the immune system reduces the risk of many illnesses.

Green Tea and Specific Diseases

Green tea polyphenols also prevent specific diseases in specific ways. For example, green tea extract has antibacterial capabilities. By damaging the membranes of bacteria, green tea polyphenols help prevent bacterial infections. Back in 1923, an army surgeon recommended that soldiers fill their water bottles with tea to prevent typhoid infections. In the days before antibiotics, this was sensible advice. In retrospect, we can conclude that boiling the water was probably more valuable than the comparatively weak antibiotic activity of the tea. Although modern research hasn't assessed the anti-typhoid potential of green tea, polyphenols have been shown to inhibit many other bacteria capable of causing infections. In particular, green tea extract prevents the growth of bacteria that cause many types of diarrhea. Researchers at the National Institute of Health in Tokyo, Japan, found that, in the laboratory, polyphenols inhibit infection by the influenza virus. In addition, green tea extract protects against disease-causing microorganisms in the gastrointestinal tract, promotes the growth of beneficial bacteria in the intestine, and may even have anti-ulcer action.[9] Although these tea effects are helpful in prevention, they are generally weaker than those of antibiotics, so a person who is sick with an infection should use antibiotics upon the advice of a health-care professional.

Green Tea and Oral Health

A number of studies based on laboratory, animal, and human evidence indicate that green tea's polyphenols are beneficial for maintaining oral health. One of the more interesting studies located thirty-five volunteers who were willing to refrain from any oral hygiene, such as brushing or flossing, for four days. Instead, these volunteers rinsed their mouths with tea extract before and after eating and before bed. Rinsing with the tea greatly reduced the deposition of cavity-promoting plaque. Other studies, which grew *Streptococcus mutans* (the bacteria responsible for dental plaque) in the laboratory, confirm that green tea polyphenols inhibit the growth of this cavity-causing bacteria.[10]

Unlocking the Secrets of Green Tea

Each day, the world's tea drinkers enjoy more than one and a half billion cups of tea. Only water is consumed in greater quantities. What is the secret to the popularity of this tasty and long-revered herb? The answer to this question surely lies in one or more of the major chemical constituents of tea, such as polyphenols, caffeine, theanine, and aromatic oils. Each plays a role in the taste, sensation, and health benefits of tea. Despite the fact that green, black, white, and oolong tea are all derived from the same plant, *Camellia sinensis,* the slightly different preparation processes used to produce each of the teas result in their distinct tastes and the slight variations in the content of active ingredients among the three types. (See "Active Ingredients in Green Tea" on the following page.)

Polyphenols

Polyphenols are naturally occurring compounds in tea that account for tea's pungency and unique flavor and have a strong antioxidant potential. The color of green tea is due in part to chlorophyll and in part to the polyphenols in tea. Exposure to oxygen during the enzymatic process

Active Ingredients in Green Tea

Following are brief descriptions of the most important active ingredients in green tea.

POLYPHENOLS

These antioxidants are the constituents in tea responsible for disease prevention and treatment. The polyphenols include epicatechin (EC), epicatechin gallate (ECG), epigallocatechin (EGC), and epigallocatechin gallate (EGCG).

CAFFEINE

This stimulant is found in tea in small amounts. Theobromine and theophylline are similar compounds also found in green tea, and they have effects similar to those of caffeine.

AROMATIC OILS

As many as five hundred different aromatic oils in tea leaves contribute to the flavor and aroma of tea.

NUTRIENTS

Tea contains vitamins (e.g., vitamin C) and minerals (e.g., fluoride and manganese). However, these nutrients are present only in very small amounts.

AMINO ACIDS (L-THEANINE)

L-theanine adds a unique quality to the taste of tea, counteracts some of the stimulant effects of caffeine, and has a relaxing effect on the body.

that is used to convert fresh tea leaves into black tea reduces polyphenol levels, giving black tea a color deeper than that of green tea and a flavor different from green tea's. The unoxidized polyphenols in green tea are responsible for its astringency, subtle color, and distinct taste. It follows that green tea and white tea, because they do not undergo oxidation, have much higher levels of unaltered polyphenols than oolong or black tea. Furthermore, since the polyphenols are the source of tea's potent health-promoting potential, it also follows that green tea (and white tea) would have the greatest effect on health—and research demonstrates that this is true. Consequently, extracts of green tea are a valuable source of the health-enhancing polyphenols.

By weight, polyphenols represent approximately 30 percent of the green tea leaf after the relatively light processing that it typically undergoes. The four primary polyphenols in green tea are:

- epicatechin (EC)
- epicatechin gallate (ECG)
- epigallocatechin (EGC)
- epigallocatechin gallate (EGCG)

These four polyphenols are often called catechins as a group. Although it can vary, one cup of green tea typically contains 142 milligrams of EGCG, 65 milligrams of EGC, 28 milligrams of ECG, and 17 milligrams of EC. Supplements of green tea extract often provide the polyphenol equivalent of up to four cups of tea or even more, and some are caffeine-free, as well.[11]

The antioxidant potential of green tea polyphenols has amazed even the scientists studying green tea. One recent study compared EGCG head-to-head with the "gold standard" of antioxidants: vitamin E. The green tea extract was shown to pack two hundred times the antioxidant punch of vitamin E.[12] And these high levels of antioxidants in the tea leaves do make it into your beverage. One study showed steeping either green or black tea for about five minutes released over 80 percent of its catechins. (This study found that instant iced tea, on the other hand, contains negligible amounts of catechins.)

At the First International Symposium on the Physiological and Pharmacological Effects of *Camellia sinensis* (Tea), Dr. Harold Graham remarked that the "scavenging effects of green tea extracts and green tea polyphenol fractions are superior to those of ascorbic acid (vitamin C) and tocopherol (vitamin E) with respect to some active oxygen radicals but are less pronounced with hydroxyl free radicals."[3] In other words, Dr. Graham had found that green tea, under some circumstances, was a more powerful antioxidant than vitamin C and vitamin E, although there are other situations where those two antioxidant vitamins are more effective than green tea. All in all, green tea makes a very impressive addition to the body's antioxidant arsenal.

Among the polyphenols found in green tea extracts, one stands out as particularly effective: EGCG. Researchers from Rutgers University, after comparing the antioxidant effect of various polyphenols in Chinese green teas and oolong tea (which is semi-oxidated), concluded that "the strong antioxidant activities of green tea are mainly due to the higher content of EGCG."[4]

Caffeine

The caffeine content of tea is the basis of tea's reputation as an uplifting and invigorating beverage. Caffeine is a central nervous system stimulant and a member of the family of chemicals called methylxanthines, which can be found in more than sixty different plants. Consumption of caffeine is widespread and popular; in fact, more than 80 percent of Americans consume at least some caffeine every day. Coffee and sodas are tied as the most frequent sources of caffeine, but about one-third of Americans drink tea regularly for their caffeine "fix." Worldwide, tea has a stronger following and accounts for 43 percent of all caffeine intake.[5]

In addition to caffeine, green, black, white, and oolong teas also contain small amounts of the methylxanthines called theobromine and theophylline. All of these methylxanthines are physiologically active, but each acts in slightly different ways in the body. Caffeine has the strongest effect on the brain and muscles, which explains the mental boost noticed shortly after drinking any caffeinated beverage. Theophylline is a powerful stimulant to the heart, respiratory system, and kidneys, which correlates with research showing that tea preserves the healthy function of the cardiovascular system. Finally, theobromine has functions similar to the other two methylxanthines, but its stimulating effects are the weakest of the three compounds. See the table on page 20 for information about the content of caffeine and theophylline in foods and beverages.

In 1827, when caffeine was first extracted from tea leaves, the substance found in tea was thought to be different from "regular" caffeine, and so it was called "theine." We now know that what researchers extracted all those years ago was in fact caffeine. Caffeine levels vary between types of tea. The auto-oxidation process increases the bioavailability of the caffeine content; therefore, black tea as a beverage contains the greatest amounts of caffeine. Oolong tea has only half the caffeine of black tea, and green tea and white tea contain only one-third the caffeine of black tea.

The effects of caffeine on the body have been well documented. And the effects of drinking tea are right in line with those of caffeine in general: Very shortly after drinking tea, there is an increase in alertness and ability to process information, as well as a mood boost. Soon after caffeine is consumed, it is completely absorbed from the gastrointestinal tract. Within an hour, caffeine levels in the bloodstream reach their peak, and caffeine remains circulating in the bloodstream for many hours. Caffeine easily crosses the blood-brain barrier and exerts effects on the brain. For instance, caffeine reduces the flow of blood to the brain by constricting the blood vessels that feed the brain. When caffeine intake is suspended, the blood vessels dilate and blood rushes to the brain, resulting in the headaches that are the primary symptom of caffeine withdrawal. Resuming caffeine consumption generally alleviates such headaches.

Caffeine has been shown in scientific studies to enhance cognitive performance, particularly for reaction time, spatial relationships, and certain aspects of memory. In addition to mental health, emotional health is affected by caffeine. It appears that caffeine staves off boredom and mental fatigue. Researchers have linked caffeine consumption with increased feelings of well-being, feeling energized, and feeling motivated to work.[16]

Caffeine has a stimulating effect on kidney function, probably because it increases blood flow to the kidneys. The respiratory system is mildly stimulated after caffeine consumption, leading to slightly faster and deeper breathing. For that reason, some asthmatics are treated with caffeine, and caffeine may help ease bronchial spasms.

Competitive athletes and weekend warriors alike dream of ergogenic

CAFFEINE AND THEOPHYLLINE CONTENT
OF FOODS AND BEVERAGES

Product (One Serving)	Caffeine	Theophylline
Coffee (brewed)	60–160 mg	0 mg
Coffee (instant)	30–120 mg	0 mg
Coffee (decaffeinated)	1–5 mg	0 mg
Soft drinks	40–70 mg	0 mg
Black tea	20–90 mg	3–4 mg
Oolong tea	10–45 mg	3–4 mg
Green tea	6–30 mg	3–4 mg
White tea	6–25 mg	3–4 mg
Tea (instant or iced)	10–45 mg	3–4 mg
Chocolate (per ounce)	1–15 mg	0 mg
Hot chocolate	2–20 mg	0 mg

aids—substances that improve physical performance. Caffeine is an ergogenic aid with relatively few harmful side effects except for people with cardiovascular disease. The research linking caffeine with enhanced athletic performance stretches back about a century. The amount of caffeine in just a few cups of tea can increase endurance and intensity during exercise. Researchers have concluded that caffeine enhances performance by increasing levels of free fatty acids in the blood; these fatty acids are then used as an energy source, sparing the body's reserves of glycogen (the storage form of glucose). The consensus of the researchers is that the ergogenic effect of caffeine is significant; it may as much as double endurance.[17]

Moderate doses of caffeine can increase the body's basal metabolic rate by approximately 10 percent. The basal metabolic rate is the amount of energy required to maintain the basic functions of breathing, pumping blood, and maintaining body temperature. This so-called thermogenic effect of caffeine, an effect that lasts about four hours, may be advantageous to weight-loss efforts. If the body is burning up more calories simply to maintain its basic functions, a person may more easily obtain a negative calorie balance and achieve weight loss. However, the potential weight-loss benefit from caffeine is minimal, especially if the beverage containing caffeine is consumed with foods containing sugar.

Several negative effects have been attributed to excessive caffeine intake. These include increased urination, diarrhea, insomnia, anxiety, heart-burn, and irritability. The amount of caffeine that leads to each of these symptoms varies with the individual. Caffeine-related insomnia shows great variation from one person to another, but, in general, the sleep-delaying effects are greatest in those who do not regularly consume caffeine. Pregnant women should steer clear of all sources of caffeine; if possible, women should even avoid caffeine entirely for a few weeks before conception. Since tea contains about half the caffeine of coffee, it is less likely to produce adverse effects. Caffeine-free supplements can be a good alternative. However, check with your physician before taking any products during pregnancy.

How sensitive a person is to caffeine is affected by many factors, including:

Body mass: The smaller you are, the quicker caffeine will affect you.
Stress: Being under stress (emotional or physical) increases sensitivity to caffeine.
History of use: If you rarely consume caffeine, you'll be more sensitive to its effects.
Medication use: Taking certain antibiotics such as ciprofloxacin (Cipro), norfloxacin (Noroxin), and enoxacin (Penetrex), the asthma medication theophylline, or the herb ephedra (ma huang), can increase the effects of caffeine.

If you want to lessen the amount of caffeine in your cup, simply brew the tea for a shorter amount of time. Of course, decaffeinated teas are another option.

The most common side effect of caffeine is probably the caffeine-withdrawal syndrome, in which symptoms of nervousness, headache, nausea, and muscle tension develop about twelve to twenty-four hours after the last ingestion of caffeine. These withdrawal symptoms are at their most severe during the second day of caffeine withdrawal and can continue for up to a week. The existence of the withdrawal syndrome would seem to suggest an addictive component of caffeine; however, research into the question of whether caffeine is addictive has been equivocal.

Excessive caffeine intake could even be lethal. A few cases of human deaths attributable to caffeine have been reported, although the circumstances were extraordinary. Evidence extrapolated from studies of animal subjects suggests that 200 caffeinated sodas, 125 cups of tea, or 75 cups of coffee consumed at one sitting would constitute a lethal dose of caffeine for a human being.

But wait, you might say, doesn't drinking tea (since it contains caffeine) dehydrate the body? While it is true that extremely high intakes of caffeine (far more than would be consumed in a few cups of tea daily) acts as a diuretic, drinking moderate amounts of tea provides you with a net gain of fluid. So rest assured that drinking tea will not leave you more dehydrated, and will instead quench your body's fluid needs.[18]

More than half of all women suffer from fibrocystic breast disease, a condition characterized by painful, lumpy breasts, at some point in their lives. The cause of fibrocystic breast disease is currently unknown, and developing this condition may coincide with an increased risk of breast cancer later in life. The role of caffeine in fibrocystic breast disease remains controversial. In the early 1980s, a study gained notoriety after finding that methylxanthines were related to the risk of developing fibrocystic breast disease. Furthermore, this study showed that as many as 65 percent of women experienced a complete alleviation of their symptoms when they eliminated coffee, tea, chocolate, and other sources of caffeine from their diets. However, later research has not confirmed any connection between caffeine and fibrocystic breast disease.

Aromatic Oils

As with polyphenol and caffeine levels, amounts of aromatic oils differ in green, black, white, and oolong teas. Aromatic oils play a large role in determining the fragrance of tea and also contribute somewhat to the taste of tea. If aromatic oils are exposed to excessive heat, they will disappear altogether, which is why they are also called volatile oils. Finely cut leaves lose their aromatic oil content more quickly than whole leaves. The aromatic oils accumulate as the tea leaf is growing and evaporate during and after the harvesting of tea leaves. Conversely, changes during the processing of tea leaves can contribute to the formation of some aromatic oils that remain in the final tea product. About five hundred different aromatic oils have been identified in some types of tea.

Vitamins and Minerals

The nutritional content of tea varies greatly according to the type of tea and the place where it was grown. Just one cup of green tea contains as much vitamin C as an entire lemon. However, vitamin C levels in black tea are much lower, since this water-soluble vitamin is partially lost during the auto-oxidation process that turns fresh tea leaves into black tea. Accordingly, green tea contains ten times the vitamin C of black tea. Despite its relatively low levels of vitamin C, black tea may have accounted for much of the vitamin C in the diets of ancient nomadic tribes in Mongolia and Central Asia, who subsisted primarily on a diet of meat and dairy products. Other vitamins found in varying amounts in tea are vitamin B_2, vitamin D, vitamin K, and the carotenoids (a family of fat-soluble pigments).

Many minerals are present in green tea, including chromium, calcium, magnesium, manganese, iron, copper, zinc, molybdenum, sodium, phosphorus, strontium, cobalt, nickel, and potassium. Depending on whether it was grown in selenium-rich or selenium-poor soil, green tea can also be a rich source of this essential mineral. Tea drinking can also be a significant source of manganese, a mineral used by the body in the digestion of protein and to maintain healthy bones and connective tissue. Just one cup of tea can provide the daily requirement of manganese.[19] The mineral content of the water used in brewing tea also contributes to the mineral content of the drink.

Although preliminary research seemed to indicate that drinking tea could interfere with the body's absorption and use of trace minerals, such as iron, and could, perhaps, increase the risk of anemia and other health concerns, further studies have shown that this is not a significant concern. One study, for example, found that even when rodents were given black tea, green tea, or a green tea extract mixed with water as their sole beverage, the risk of anemia was not increased. When it is necessary to take non-hemic ferrous salt iron supplements, it is prudent to take them one hour before or two hours after consuming tea. But keep in mind that there is no reason for healthy people who have no risk factors for anemia to restrict their tea consumption.

Tea, and green tea in particular, is also an impressive source of fluoride—the mineral well known for fighting cavities. Many communities add fluoride to their water supplies in order to take advantage of its dental benefits. These supplies of fluoridated water generally provide 0.7 to 1.2 parts per million of fluoride. In contrast, many teas provide 1.32 to 4.18 parts per million of fluoride. Research into the dental benefits of green tea confirms that green tea does, in fact, reduce the incidence of dental cavities, although researchers believe that the catechins are primarily responsible for the anticaries effect.[20]

There has been some concern about the seemingly high levels of the mineral aluminum found in tea, particularly since an excessive intake of aluminum may be associated with serious bone and brain disorders. However, researchers have discovered that aluminum is present in tea in a complex, rather than ionic, form, which is less absorbable and has much less potential to have an adverse effect on health. Studies conducted on animals show that frequent consumption of green tea does not contribute significantly to the body's aluminum burden, nor does the mineral accumulate in the bones. One researcher concluded that concerns about any deleterious effects of aluminum from tea are "unfounded"[21]

Amino Acids

Green tea contains several amino acids (the building blocks of proteins) including aspartic acid, glutamic acid, glycine, serine, glutamine, tyrosine, threonine, alanine, valine, leucine, isoleucine, phenylalanine, lysine, arginine, histidine, tryptophan, aspargine, and proline. Besides these common amino acids, green tea contains another amino acid that is unique to it: theanine. Theanine constitutes about half of the total amino acid levels in green tea, and its presence is said to correlate with tea quality. All of the amino acids are involved in the formation of tea's aroma; however, the unique amino acid, theanine, is reputed to be one of the tastier components of green tea. Theanine accounts for more than half of the free amino acid content of green tea, and also plays a role in the biosynthesis of polyphenols. Theanine has caught the eye of cancer r〔 〕 since this green tea extract enhances the effectiveness of some 〔 〕 medications while minimizing their side effects.

L-theanine is made in the roots of the tea plant, and then travels to the leaves. (L-theanine is chemically derived from the more common amino acid glutamic acid.) Once in the leaves, some of this amino acid is converted (after exposure to sunlight) into polyphenols. Some tea cultivators, who want to preserve higher levels of L-theanine, for flavor purposes, grow their tea plants out of direct sunlight.

Most amino acids do not cross over into the brain; however, L-theanine does and once there it counteracts some of the stimulant effects of caffeine. Once in the brain, L-theanine interacts with receptors that are associated with relaxation, resulting in a relaxed but alert state of mind. Its ability to promote relaxation without leading to drowsiness is accounted for by changes in levels of serotonin, dopamine, and other neurotransmitters. In one study of university students, taking 200 milligrams of L-theanine eased anxiety and increased alpha brain wave activity after forty minutes; alpha brain waves are the type associated with relaxation.[22] Other benefits noted in laboratory and animal research from L-theanine include lower blood pressure, improved learning ability, and even a boost to the infection-fighting immune system.

Supplements of L-theanine are very safe, with no reported side effects or adverse reactions. You can take it in the amount of 200 milligrams once or twice a day and you might feel an improved sense of well-being within an hour of taking it.

Green tea is certainly in a class unto itself in terms of the diverse ways it supports good health. Almost every system of the body is beneficially affected by green tea, since green tea lowers cholesterol and blood pressure, which reduces the risk of heart attack and stroke; prevents cancer from starting and spreading; boosts immunity and fights infection; and even helps prevent dental cavities. In the following chapters, all of these health benefits will be explored in greater detail, but first we will explore the history of this interesting beverage.

chapter two

The "Hottest" Historic Beverage

Tea is the most popular beverage, after water, throughout the world. Not surprisingly, there is a rich mythology surrounding the history of tea and its important role in many cultures around the world.

While a "nice cup of tea" is inextricably linked to our modern concept of tea, not all cultures have made a cup of tea in the same way or even served it in a cup. In fact, the archeological record indicates that wild tea may first have been used as a food, not a beverage. In Thailand, steamed tea leaves were formed into balls and eaten with salt, oil, garlic, pig fat, and dried fish; in parts of India, tea was combined with red potash, anise seeds, and salt; ancient Burmese people pickled tea leaves and used them as a salad; and in Tibet, tea was made into a breakfast meal by adding barley, salt, and goat's milk butter and churning it until it reached a creamy consistency. In this chapter, we'll take a look at the history of tea throughout the world's cultures. (See "Milestones in the History of Tea" on page 28.)

Tea Is Discovered

Myths and legends obscure the discovery of tea, but we know without a doubt that wild tea plants originated throughout Southeast Asia, particularly in China. The first written references to tea date from about 3000 B.C., although tea was undoubtedly used much earlier than that.

Milestones in the History of Tea

Tea's history begins in China thousands of years ago. This chart outlines the key events in tea's progress to its present worldwide popularity.

Tea Time	Event
2737 B.C.	A Chinese medical book includes the earliest known written reference to tea as a health aid.
A.D. 350	A Chinese dictionary describes the method for making tea.
479	Turkish traders barter for tea at the Mongolian border.
500	Another Chinese dictionary includes an entry describing tea as a pleasant beverage.
520	According to legend, Bodhidharma, a Buddhist monk, tears off his eyelids to punish himself for falling asleep during meditation, and a tea plant sprouts from where they land.
350–600	Chinese tea cultivation techniques are improved by Chinese farmers trying to meet the growing demand for tea.
780	Lu Yu writes the *Ch'a Ching (Book of Tea)*.
794	The Japanese emperor creates a government post to tend tea plants, an indication of the importance of tea.
850	*An Account of Tea by Two Arabian Travelers* is published and further acquaints the Western world with Chinese tea.
1211	A small book about tea published in Japan increases tea's popularity in that country.

Tea Time	Event
1333	A tea-drinking game, called tocha, reaches height of popularity in Japan.
Circa 1450	The Japanese tea ceremony is formalized by Murata Shuko.
1517	Portuguese sailors arrive in China and trade for tea.
1559	*Voyages and Travels,* published in Europe, discusses the health benefits of tea.
1606	The Dutch East India Company imports first shipment of Chinese tea to Europe.
1618	Czar Alexis of Russia receives a gift of Chinese tea.
1635	The first reports of Europeans drinking tea.
1657	Tea is available for purchase by the British public.
1660	The British government levies tax on importation of tea.
1834	The first attempt is made to cultivate Chinese tea in India.
1848	Robert Fortune, a British adventurer, pretends to be a Chinese merchant in order to learn the secrets of Chinese tea cultivation.
1869	The coffee crop in Ceylon (now Sri Lanka) is decimated by fungus. Tea crops are grown as a replacement and become an important export product for this country.
1904	Iced tea introduced at the St. Louis World's Fair.
Today	Tea's popularity continues to grow as scientific research details the health benefits of this beverage.

According to one of the most well-known tea myths, Emperor Shen Nong (who lived at about the same time as Moses) believed that boiling water before drinking it was a key to continued good health. While he was boiling water in his garden, a leaf from a nearby bush wafted into his pot. Rather than remove the wayward leaf, he allowed it to brew in the water, and he drank the resulting liquid. He was pleased with this decoction and declared it to have even more healing power than boiled water alone. This myth coincides with evidence showing that early use of tea involved boiling wild tea leaves in water. Another myth of the origin of tea tells the tale of Bodhidharma (sometimes called Daruma), an Indian monk who founded the Japanese school of Buddhism. According to this story, around A.D. 520 Bodhidharma was traveling from India to China. When he arrived in Canton, he was offered sanctuary in a temple cave in the mountains near the capital of the Chinese Emperor Liang Wu Ti. Bodhidharma vowed to stay awake and meditate for nine years, but he fell asleep after only a few years. When he awoke, he was so upset at his weakness that he cut off his eyelids and threw them angrily to the ground. A tea plant soon took root and grew from the spot where his bloody eyelids had landed, to serve as a reminder of Bodhidharma's weakness and sacrifice. Zen monks recommended chewing the eyelid-shaped leaves of this plant to maintain alertness during Zen meditation, making the leaves a highly valued commodity.

Of course the legend of Bodhidharma is allegorical, but experts have pointed out that chewing tea leaves was already an established practice around the time this legend is supposed to have taken place. Other archeological evidence even suggests that *Homo erectus pekinensis* added various herbs (presumably including tea leaves) to boiling water 500,000 years before any of these tea myths were developed or modern man even existed.

Following the written record, tea does not turn up again until the twelfth century B.C., when tribal leaders in China included tea in their tributes to the founder of the Zhou Dynasty. Tracing the history of tea in Chinese culture is difficult for two reasons. First, the Chinese character for tea has changed over the centuries. The modern character "ch'a" has been used only since the seventh century A.D. Before then, the symbol "t'u" was used interchangeably to refer both to tea and to another herb, the sow thistle. Consequently, it is hard to determine in early records which herb is being discussed. The second difficulty in tracing the history of tea arises from the fact that whenever a new Chinese dynasty came into power, it was common procedure for the new ruling emperor to distort previously accepted historical accounts. If the members of the new dynasty wished to credit themselves for the discovery of tea, they would.

The first reference to the cultivation of tea appeared in A.D. 350, in Kuo P'o's updated version of an ancient Chinese dictionary, the *Erh Ya*, first written in the eighteenth century B.C. Kuo P'o's added entry about tea explains that "a beverage is made from the leaves by boiling." Tea was primarily used during this era of history as a cure for digestive and nervous disorders, although it was also used as a salve to cure rheumatic pain. Another dictionary, the *Kuang Ya*, written in A.D. 500, described tea as a pleasing beverage. At that time, tea beverages were primarily prepared by boiling tea leaves in water and adding onion, ginger, and orange.

Besides its use as a food, beverage, stimulant, and medicine, tea had other uses in ancient China. Tribal people living in the interior of China would compress bricks of tea with primitive ox-presses and use these tea bricks as currency to exchange with other tribes. It is interesting to note that in ancient cultures the value of minted money generally decreased the farther one was from the place where it had been minted. In contrast, tea bricks, as currency, increased in value the farther one traveled from the place where they had been made, since tea was cultivated only in limited areas and was a rare commodity beyond those areas.

Tea Becomes an Art in China

The demand for tea began to increase dramatically between A.D. 350 and A.D. 600. Before then, farmers had gathered tea leaves by cutting down wild tea trees thirty feet tall and stripping the branches of their leaves. With the increasing demand for tea, the wild tea trees were in danger of being eradicated. To ensure ongoing tea crops, a group of farmers banded together to develop more effective ways to cultivate tea. They decided what kind of soil was best for growing tea plants and chose the Szechwan district as the first tea-growing area because its soil and hilly terrain met their requirements.

Demand continued to soar. Even with new sources of cultivated tea, farmers were having trouble keeping China's thirsty teapots filled. Soon tea farmers began growing tea plants in the Yangtze valley and along the coast. The increasing attention paid to tea in Chinese culture is epitomized by the *Ch'a Ching* or *Book of Tea*, written by Lu Yu in A.D. 780. This classic three-volume book covered the proper techniques for growing, preparing, and brewing tea and helped earn Lu Yu a place in Chinese history as the "patron saint" of tea. Lu Yu's exhaustive description of the best way to prepare tea, in which he mentions twenty-four utensils, later formed the basis of the Japanese tea ceremony.

According to Chinese beliefs, certain people can be elevated to divine rank after their deaths because in life they were models of excellence or benefited the human race. Lu Yu was honored with this immortal status because of his life work in promoting tea.

Lu Yu's life story is very interesting, although much of it is undocumented. As a baby, he was abandoned beside a river in central China. Luckily, he was found and adopted by a Buddhist abbot from the Dragon Cloud Monastery, and subsequently given the name Lu Yu, which was derived from a line of text in the *I Ching*. However, when he refused to become a monk, his adoptive father punished him by giving him drudgery to do, including the job of cleaning the monastery's bathrooms. Instead, Lu Yu ran off with a traveling entertainment troupe. Later, he settled down in a province of China renowned for its scholars and spent the rest of his life writing scholarly works, such as the *Ch'a Ching*.

After writing his definitive work on tea, Lu Yu was befriended by the Emperor himself. Through the renown that the Emperor's patronage brought him, Lu Yu attracted an entourage of disciples who closely followed his guidelines for making tea. Some tea aficionados even claimed to be able to distinguish tea brewed by the master himself from that merely made by his followers.

Even Lu Yu's adoptive father was singularly impressed with his son's tea brewing. Apparently, father and son reunited at some point, because Lu Yu returned to the monastery, only to leave it again. After Lu Yu left the monastery for the second time, his father refused to drink tea again, since the tea offered to him was not made by his son's expert hand. The Emperor, hearing this interesting tale, decided to test the abbot's taste for tea and invited him to the capital. When he arrived, the Emperor offered him tea brewed by a lady of the court who was reputed to be among the most capable in the art of tea. The abbot, out of respect, tried the tea, but then set it aside. The Emperor, expecting to trick the abbot, then had Lu Yu secretly brought to the palace where he was commanded to brew tea for an unnamed guest. Again the abbot tried the tea, but this time he drank it contentedly and declared "Now this tea is superb, not even my son could do better!" The Emperor, now convinced of Lu Yu's special tea skills and the abbot's discriminating palate, brought father and son together for another reunion.

Another story about Lu Yu's legendary tea-making abilities concerns the water he used. In Lu Yu's time, the water with which tea was brewed was of the utmost importance, and tasting the fine distinctions between water from various sources was a central part of the tea art. On a trip down the Yangtze River, Lu Yu spent some time as a guest of a high-ranking dignitary. While visiting, he was asked to taste a jar of water drawn from the center of the river, which was said to be the cleanest and tastiest. After taking a small sip, Lu Yu, with disgust, declared it to be low-quality water drawn near the bank of the river. The man responsible for drawing the water denied that it was from near the bank of the river, so Lu Yu took another sip. He then conceded that it could be water drawn from midstream, but it must have been diluted with inferior water. At this point, the man admitted that while he was returning to shore some of the water he had drawn from the center of the river had spilled and he had replaced the lost quantity with water from near the river bank. The man added "Master Lu, you are clearly an Immortal!"

One of Lu Yu's disciples was Lu T'ung, whose passion for tea is evident in his nickname, which can be loosely translated as "tea maniac." Lu T'ung devoted his life to poetry and the preparation of tea. He is remembered for writing a poem that includes the line: "I am in no way interested in immortality, but only in the taste of tea."

Tea Spreads from the Elite to the Populace

At about the time that the *Ch'a Ching* was written, we find the first recorded use of a "tea tax." Apparently, Lu Yu had raved about the quality of tea from a certain region; in response, an imperial envoy was dispatched to bring back a small quantity as a sample. The court so enjoyed this fine tea that the emperor demanded that the region send an annual supply as a "tribute." Over time, this tribute inflated to thousands of pounds each year, with all the tea-producing regions subject to the tea tribute. It eventually became quite a burden to the peasants in the tea-cultivating provinces. Historians estimate that thirty thousand peasants were involved in picking and processing tea during the harvesting season (a thirty-day period each year) just to meet the tribute demand.

The exact day to start the harvest was selected by tea officials who gathered at mountain temples and made sacrifices to a mountain deity. Very early in the morning on the appointed day, the tea pickers, who were mostly young girls, would be sent up the mountain slopes, where the tea crops grew, to gather the tea leaves at their peak. Picking stopped each day at noon, when the processing of the tea leaves began and continued until sunset.

Over the next few hundred years (especially during the reign of the Sung Dynasty from 960 to 1127), tea drinking rose to an art form. Tearooms and teahouses developed as social and spiritual gathering places. One of the emperors of the Sung Dynasty, Hui Tsung, even became known as the "Tea Emperor" after his love of tea inspired him to write a treatise on tea.

The harvesting of tea became even more closely regulated during this dynasty. Drum and cymbal signals were used to coordinate the tea pickers in the fields during the chilly, dark pre-dawn hours. The girls received training as tea pickers and even wore identification labels on their jackets so that tea thieves could be more readily spotted if they entered the tea estates. The girls were instructed to keep their fingernails at a precise length, since the nails, never the fingers, were used to pluck the highest quality tea leaves.

The freshly picked leaves were graded into classes and processed. The best grades of tea were delivered as tribute tea, and the rest were traded and sold by the regional government. The values placed on the top grades of tea were impressive. A cake of high-grade tea (a quantity that could easily be held in the palm of a hand) might be worth as much as two ounces of gold, while the very choicest grades were simply beyond price.

Emperor Hui Tsung's search for the perfect cup of tea took him beyond even the strict harvesting guidelines of this era. His "imperial plucking" method dictated that tea leaves destined for his tea cup be picked only by young virgins wearing gloves and wielding gold scissors with which to shear the delicate tips from the leaves of the tea plants.

During the Sung Dynasty the art of making beautiful ceramics—which were used as tea accessories—was perfected. Prior to this era, people drank tea from bowls, but in this dynasty the bowls were replaced with saucer-like vessels called *chien*. The tea connoisseurs of this dynasty established tea contests to test their tea-brewing prowess, competing against one another to brew the finest tea, which judges assessed for several qualities, including the original quality of the tea leaves, the purity of the water, and the taste of the final product.

This peaceful era of tea appreciation did not last. In the early part of the thirteenth century, Mongolian invaders, under such infamous leaders as Genghis Khan and Kublai Khan, conquered a growing number of Chinese territories, eventually establishing a Mongolian dynasty that remained in power for more than a century. For the first time in centuries, the Chinese government and China's social elite no longer showed interest in tea. In fact, when Marco Polo arrived in China in 1275, he was not even introduced to tea. Tea was "rediscovered" when the Chinese regained power over their own country after a hundred-fifty years of Mongolian rule, but this time, tea was not an elixir for the elite alone to drink; it was transformed into a beverage to be enjoyed daily by the entire populace, as it is today.

Tea Thrives in Japan

During the lean years of Mongolian rule in tea's Chinese history (from 1206 to 1368), Japan kept the appreciation and traditions of tea alive. Actually, tea had been introduced to Japan long before this. Records show that tea was already known and appreciated by 729, when the emperor gave gifts of powdered tea to a hundred monks attending a Buddhist scripture reading at the palace. Many of these monks began to cultivate tea upon returning to their temples. In 794, Emperor Kammu moved the capital and built a new palace, taking the opportunity to build an enclosed tea garden at the palace. He then decided to create a new government post for an official to tend the tea plants: Supervisor of the Tea Gardens. The fact that this new post was within the medical bureau of the government reveals Japan's respect for the curative potential of tea.

For the next few centuries, Japan was dependent on China both for imported supplies of tea and for the culture surrounding the preparation and enjoyment of tea. Because tea arrived from China in limited quantities and Japan did not grow very much of its own, tea became a luxury used for medicinal and spiritual purposes only by the upper classes. This quality of preciousness probably contributed to the later development of the Japanese tea ceremony.

The man who founded Zen Buddhism in Japan, Eisai Myoan, traveled to China during the years 1187 to 1191 in order to study Chinese philosophy. When he returned to his home country of Japan, he brought tea seeds with him and planted them on the grounds of his temple. Eisai soon realized that this new tea was far superior to the tea that had previously been growing in Japan. Inspired by this higher quality tea, he experimented with different ways to brew it. At that time, most people in Japan boiled tea leaves in water, but Eisai found that grinding the leaves into a powder and mixing that with hot water enhanced the flavor of the resulting drink.

After years of perfecting the growth and preparation of tea, Eisai wrote a small book on tea in 1211, the title of which loosely translates to *Tea Drinking Is Good for Health*. In this book he wrote that drinking tea confers many benefits, including curing lack of appetite, diseases caused by poor quality drinking water, paralysis, boils, and beri-beri (a B-vitamin deficiency). Eisai went so far as to claim that tea was a remedy for almost all health problems.

Eisai's confidence in the healing properties of tea was soon put to the test. A government official who was in danger of dying from the ill effects of gluttony asked Eisai to pray for his recovery. Rather than trusting this man's fate solely to the power of prayer, Eisai directed the official to drink tea that Eisai himself had cultivated and prepared. After the official recovered, Eisai gave him a copy of his book, and the official became a strong tea supporter. As the amazing story of tea's contribution to this man's recovery from deathly illness spread, demand for and cultivation of tea increased throughout the island country of Japan.

Around this time, another tea enthusiast developed the "Ten Virtues of Tea" and inscribed them on a tea kettle. The ten virtues are as follows:

1. Has the blessing of all the Deities.
2. Promotes filial piety.
3. Drives away the Devil.

4. Banishes drowsiness.
5. Keeps the Five Viscera in harmony.
6. Wards off disease.
7. Strengthens friendships.
8. Disciplines body and mind.
9. Destroys the passions.
10. Gives a peaceful death.

Throughout the 1200s, tea drinking continued to grow in popularity in Japan, particularly in the emerging samurai class, but it was not until 1333, when several civil wars broke out and a new class of elite came into power, that tea reached a new height of popularity in Japan. One offshoot of this was a game called *tocha*, which was based on the tea-drinking contests that had developed in China more than a century earlier. This game started out as a "test" for guests at a party to distinguish genuine tea from fake tea made from herbs with a taste similar to tea. As farmers began to grow tea in more places around the country, the game evolved to become a test of skill in identifying tea strains, the part of the country in which the tea had been grown, and even the name of the plantation where a particular tea had been cultivated. As the game became more complicated, prizes were added as incentive for competition. All classes of people enjoyed this game, and the most elite classes would sometimes raise the stakes as high as a hundred rolls of dyed silk to be awarded to the winner.

Of course, the drinking of tea was the basis of these games. Initially, each guest was served about ten cups of tea at these gatherings, but as the games grew more complex, each guest could be served as many as a hundred cups of tea at a party that started early in the morning and lasted into the middle of the night. It is very likely that each cup of tea was passed from guest to guest and shared, rather than dozens of cups being placed in front of each guest. By the time the civil wars ended and Ashikaga Takauji established leadership at the end of the fourteenth century, the tea games had gotten so out of control that he banned them. Despite the ban, many people continued to enjoy tea games, particularly soldiers and peasants. Even priests continued to play the game.

Preparing and serving tea was also an important part of entertaining guests in this era. Most well-to-do Japanese families, especially those of

the samurai class, set aside certain rooms in their house for the purpose of entertaining their guests with tea. These Japanese homes were
decorated with imported Chinese artwork, and their owners prepared
tea with imported Chinese utensils. Many Japanese hosts partitioned
off small areas of larger rooms to be used for tea entertainment, since
they felt that smaller rooms were more comfortable and less formal for
their guests. As this partitioning became more popular, Japanese build-
ers began to design and build smaller rooms expressly for serving tea;
this style of entertaining became the basis for the famous Japanese tea
ceremony.

Tea Inspires a Ceremony

The father of the Japanese tea ceremony was a Zen priest named Murata
Shuko (1422–1502). He first became well known as an accomplished
designer of the smaller tearooms popular in Japan at that time. Shuko
enjoyed the intimacy of serving tea in a small room. In fact, he established the four-and-a-half-mat room size, which was literally formed by
tatami mats fitted together to define the area of the tearoom. He felt that
a room this size encouraged a more tranquil atmosphere. Others of his
era would have servants serve tea, as a sign of their wealth, but Shuko
felt that having the host serve the guests was an integral part of the tea-
sharing experience.

Shuko's interest in tea began somewhat accidentally. He had entered
the priesthood at eleven years of age, but he was expelled for laziness.
He began studying under a learned master, but again his tendency to
fall asleep during the day threatened the success of his endeavors. He
consulted a doctor for advice on how to stay awake; the doctor told him
that he should drink tea frequently to stimulate his mind. Shuko found
tea-drinking to be a very successful method of maintaining his mental
clarity; he drank tea frequently and offered it to others.

Shuko devoted his life to drinking and preparing tea, eventually developing the Japanese tea ceremony. The guidelines of Shuko's tea ceremony
have been preserved in a letter he wrote to his favorite student, Harima
no Furuichi. Repeatedly, Shuko wrote about the importance of refined
simplicity as an integral aspect of tea appreciation. Eventually, Shuko's
interpretation of the Japanese tea ceremony would become the definitive

way to practice the tea ceremony. It was named *chanoyu*, which literally means "hot water for tea."

Devotees of the tea ceremony say that there are two types of tea masters: those who treasure the formality and beauty of the ceremony, its atmosphere, and its utensils, and those who love the spirituality of the ceremony. A respected tea master, Sen Rikyu, was once asked by one of his disciples what should be kept in mind during the tea ceremony. Rikyu responded: "Tea is not difficult. Suggest coolness in summer and warmth in winter. Set the charcoal so that the water will boil. The flowers should be arranged as if they were still in the field."

As a tea master of wide renown, Rikyu adapted and perfected several of the aspects of the tea ceremony founded by Shuko. His outstanding contributions to the Japanese tea ceremony earned him an invitation in 1585 to become the tea master at the Imperial Palace. However, with this new power, Rikyu began to act arrogantly and insolently. Because of this behavior and rumors circulating about him, the emperor ordered him to commit suicide, which he did on February 28, 1591.

The goal of the Japanese tea ceremony is for the host and guests to attain spiritual satisfaction through the drinking of tea and quiet contemplation of the tearoom. The Japanese tea ceremony is a blend of many influences, particularly Zen philosophy and the Chinese custom of drinking tea. Each tea ceremony is designed to be a singular experience, although a strict protocol is followed. Everything associated with the tea ceremony is meaningful, from the architecture of the buildings in which the tea is served and the design of the utensils used to prepare the tea to the host's presentation of the tea. The strong Zen basis for the Japanese tea ceremony results from the fact that most of the early tea masters were priests from the Zen religion. Zen followers believe that enlightenment is attained through meditation, and the tea ceremony was seen as a way to discipline the mind for meditation. In fact, a well-known saying claims that "tea and Zen are one and the same."

What was originally a "tearoom" set aside within a house later became a separate building called the *sukiya* or teahouse, which consisted of four parts: the *mizu-ya*, or anteroom, used for storing the tea utensils; the *machi-ai*, a waiting room located a short distance away from the tea chamber, where the guests (rarely more than five) wait to be summoned by the host; the *roji*, a path that connects the waiting room to the tea room; and the tearoom, which is distinguished by its simplicity, where the actual ceremony is conducted. The tea served at the ceremony is a bright green powdered tea called *matcha*, which is made from pulverized green tea leaves.

When summoned from the waiting room by the host, the guests walk along the path thinking reverently about the ceremony and then enter the tearoom by crawling through a low doorway. This unusual entrance to the tearoom is considered a way of humbling guests of all ranks and making all of the guests equal. The only decorations in the tearoom itself are usually a single monochrome painting or painted scroll and a flower arrangement, which the guests pause to admire. Delicately scented incense wafts through the tearoom. The guests are offered a light meal. After a ritual involving the serving and eating of this meal, the guests return to the waiting room while the host cleans up the remains of the meal and prepares the tea. At the sound of a gong, the guests return to the tearoom and watch the host heat a kettle of water and whisk green tea powder into water in a bowl and transform it into a thick tea. Each guest tastes the tea, praises the flavor, wipes the rim of the bowl, and passes it to the next guest. The host then makes a second batch of tea, this one a thin tea, which is served in individual tea bowls. The host then leaves the tearoom, taking all of the tea utensils away, and the ceremony is concluded.

Tea Arrives in Europe

The record of what may have been the Western world's earliest experience with tea has been preserved in Chinese writings but, apparently, not by any Western historians. It seems that in A.D. 479, Turkish traders arrived on the Mongolian border and bartered for tea, but we have no record of tea's reception back in Turkey. The next recorded Western contact with tea occurred in 850, when a man named Suleiman wrote *An Account of Tea by Two Arabian Travelers.* Exposure to Chinese tea outside Asia remained minimal over the next few centuries, until Portuguese mariners reached China in the year 1517.

Before the Portuguese established a sea route around Africa to China, Venice was the commercial center to which traders brought treasures from the Orient to be exchanged for European goods. In addition to silks, dyes, and spices, traders began to bring tea to Venice. Hajji Mahommed, a Persian merchant, shared stories about tea with Gaimbattista Ramusio, the secretary to the Venetian Council of Ten. Ramusio included information about the health-enhancing properties of tea in his 1559 book *Voyages and Travels*. This was the first mention of tea in a European book.

Venice's monopoly on trade was short-lived. The overland routes that brought foreign goods to Venice took a long time to travel and were very treacherous, so, when the Portuguese successfully developed a sea route based on Vasco de Gama's explorations, they were able to dominate trade with the Orient, since their goods were cheaper. The Chinese allowed the Portuguese to build a trading center on Macao, a peninsula and two accompanying islands in the Canton River, but European traders and explorers were not allowed to go into the Chinese mainland. Missionaries, however, did reach the interior, and many of them later provided accounts of the use of tea. Father Gaspar da Cruz, a Portuguese Jesuit, wrote in 1560 about the "bitter, red, and medicinal" drink of tea. Father Matteo Ricci, who became the scientific adviser to the Chinese court, wrote in the early 1600s that he believed tea drinking was the basis of Chinese longevity.

In 1606, the Dutch East India Company imported the first shipments of tea from China. The trading company acquired three measures of tea for each measure of sage exchanged. The crews of the trading ships of that era had a hard life. Three out of four sailors never made it back home, mostly as a result of scurvy and infectious diseases. Ironically, many more might have made it back home alive if they had drunk their cargo instead of just transporting it. The vitamin C in green tea prevents scurvy, and tea's polyphenols boost the body's immune function so that it can better fight infectious disease.

By the 1630s, each Dutch vessel returning to Europe from China routinely carried several large pottery jars of tea. Accordingly, there are records of people drinking tea in Amsterdam, London, and Paris as early as 1635. A Dutch physician, Cornelius Bontekoe, even advised everyone to drink eight to ten cups of tea daily, adding that he saw no reason not to drink as many as a hundred cups daily. (It should be noted that the cups commonly used for tea drinking at that time were quite small.) Interestingly enough, based on modern research, his recommendation about how much tea would preserve good health was not too far off the mark. At this stage of history, tea was still an expensive luxury in Europe, enjoyed primarily by high society. Tea reached the general British public in 1657, when it was first offered for public sale at Garway's Coffee House in London. Garway informed his customers that drinking tea "vanquisheth heavy dreams, easeth the Brain, and strengtheneth the Memory." These claims may at first glance seem like hyperbole, but modern research is proving that many of the early claims for tea were basically true.

The British government, taking advantage of tea's growing popularity, levied a tax on imported tea in 1660. This tax remained in place until the 1780s, although many Englishmen, having become voracious in their appetite for tea, found ways around the tax. Servants in well-to-do homes would dry used tea leaves and resell them; some peddlers cut tea leaves with herbs—such as beech, hawthorn, and logwood—to extend their stock; and smugglers worked hard to find creative ways to sneak tea into the country, thereby avoiding the tax.

Clearly, not everyone exposed to tea understood its use and value. When a Scottish household was sent a pound of tea by the widow of the duke of Monmouth, the cook—who hadn't been told how to prepare this delicacy—boiled the tea leaves, tossed out the water, and served the leaves like a dish of spinach. It didn't take long, however, for British households to learn the art of brewing and drinking tea.

Meanwhile, China maintained its monopoly of the tea market. Most of the tea arriving on British shores made it there by way of the East India Company, which was chartered in 1599 with Queen Elizabeth's approval. In the early days, tea was only an incidental commodity, while silk, coffee, and spices powered this trading company. However, the English were destined to become one of the most tea-loving countries, and they soon expanded the importation of tea. By 1669, the East India Company was importing tea from China regularly. In that year, about 150 pounds of tea was shipped to England. Just a few years later, in 1705, the yearly import of tea grew to approximately 800,000 pounds. England's passion for tea continued to grow, and by the 1850s England's tea drinkers were consuming more than 80 million pounds of tea annually.

By the early eighteenth century, many Europeans recognized the healing properties of tea. The French Cardinal Mazarin believed that drinking tea helped treat his gout, and Samuel Pepys recorded in his diary that drinking tea brought his wife relief from colds and bronchitis. But not everyone was a tea enthusiast. In 1678, Henry Saville denounced tea drinking, and in 1756 Jonas Hanway claimed in his *Essay on Tea* that drinking tea spoiled the good looks of both men and women. At one time there was even a rumor circulating through Europe that tea sapped a person's vitality and that the Chinese exported it in order to weaken their enemies. One can find no modern support for these peculiar beliefs.

In the mid-nineteenth century, driven by England's ravenous appetite for tea and the demand for fresher tea, merchants began to experiment with faster ways to bring tea to the marketplace. These experiments led to the birth of the great clipper ship era. Clipper ships were slim, sleek vessels with several masts and vast expanses of billowing sails that gathered every gust of wind. This new class of sailing ship reduced the travel time along the tea-trade route from months to weeks; some clippers made the trip from Hong Kong to London in as short a time as ninety-five days.

Famous clipper ship races were held, with various trading companies vying to be the first to bring a new harvest of tea to the marketplace. The great era of stately clipper ships was short-lived. It ended in 1869, when the Suez Canal opened, shortening the trip to China and making less glamorous steamships the more economical way to transport tea to British teapots.

Tea Reaches the Rest of the World

While tea was entering Europe and England via ocean routes, Russians were acquiring their taste for tea through the dangerous and laborious overland route. As early as 1567, a couple of Cossacks had told stories about the Chinese drink, but tea did not officially arrive in Russia until 1618, when Czar Alexis received the generous gift of several chests of tea from Chinese ambassadors. Trading caravans were established in 1689, with three hundred camels traveling 11,000 miles from Russia to China and back over the course of sixteen months. The route took the caravan through Mongolia and the Gobi desert, with each camel carrying 600 pounds of tea. To lighten the burden of this much tea, the caravans did not store the tea in heavy chests, as the sea-traders did, but stuffed the tea leaves into cloth sacks. Over the long journey, the tea leaves were imbued with the scent of nightly campfires, and this smoky flavor became the hallmark of Russian Caravan tea. Also, since ceramic teapots were too fragile to survive the long journey, the metallic samovar developed as a sensible way to prepare water for tea, and remains popular in Russian culture.

Tea drinking also became a popular pastime in parts of Africa. In Egypt, people have been drinking black tea since the fifteenth century, and in Morocco, green tea mixed with mint has been a popular drink since British traders introduced it about a hundred years ago. Some African countries have even begun to grow tea; they include Kenya, Cameroon, and South Africa.

The history of tea in the Americas is colorful. Some historians suggest that Dutch settlers may have brought tea to New Amsterdam (later to become New York) before it was introduced in England. Tea remained a popular beverage with the British colonists. In 1773, however, America's relationship with tea took a turn for the worse. A group of colonists known as the Sons of Liberty, incensed by what they regarded as excessive taxation by the British government, dressed up as Indians and emptied the cargo of tea chests from the East India Company's ships moored in Boston Harbor, a cargo that would be valued at more than $200 million today. England was annoyed. One of the officially stated purposes of the tax was to pay for the maintenance of troops to protect the colonists and to maintain order. Whose version of the dispute was more correct would probably not be of much interest today if the Boston Tea Party had not become one of the events that led to the American Revolution. Tea has traveled a long, slow road back to its former level of appreciation in the new United States.

Today tea is found in almost 80 percent of all U.S. households. On any given day, about half of Americans (127 million of them) drink tea, with about 87 percent of it being black, 12.5 percent green, and the rest oolong or white. In all, in one recent year, Americans were found to have consumed over 2.25 billion gallons of tea. A drink called chai (which is a mixture of black tea, milk, and spices) that originated in India has become popular in the United States and other parts of the world.

Tea Is Grown Outside of China

Wild tea plants grow in Northern India, but for most of history, Chinese tea has been the only tea cultivated for widespread use. China was able to maintain its exclusive status as the exporter of tea because it restricted all knowledge of tea cultivation techniques. The British, eager to learn the secrets of tea, acquired several thousand tea seeds in 1834 and sent them to nurseries in Calcutta, India. There they discovered that just having tea seeds did not result in a high-quality finished product; special cultivation and processing methods are the secret to producing tasty tea. Consequently, the British government sent a man named Robert Fortune to China in 1848 to uncover the secrets of growing tea. He disguised himself as a Chinese merchant and traveled with two Chinese companions. Fortune traveled very discreetly, mostly at night, but managed to study tea plantations and keep a detailed journal, taking particular regard of proper soils, plucking techniques, and the processing of the tea leaves. All of this knowledge had been carefully guarded from foreigners, and no foreigner had previously managed to learn it.

Seeds gathered by Fortune were later given to British colonists in an attempt to establish tea plantations in India; these efforts generally failed. However, other experiments, which involved clearing the Indian jungle, planting native tea plants, and cultivating them with the Chinese techniques Fortune had learned, were much more successful.

At the time, few people suspected that the island of Ceylon (now Sri Lanka), a British colony that was famous for its coffee, would also become a well-known tea producing region, but that is just what happened in the mid-1800s. The shift from coffee to tea occurred in 1869 when the coffee crop was wiped out by an invasion of a deadly fungus. With the coffee crop in ruins, the plantation owners looked for a way to save the island's economy and found that tea was just the replacement they needed. Since then, tea has remained an important export product for Sri Lanka.

Today leading tea producing countries include Argentina, Brazil, China, India, Indonesia, Kenya, Malawi, Sri Lanka, and Tanzania.

It's clear, from the rich history of tea, that this wonderful beverage was too enjoyable to remain confined to just one corner of the world. Today, tea is cherished as a stimulating morning pick-me-up, a soothing ritual in the afternoon, and a great way to support a healthy life in virtually every country of the world.

chapter three

Antioxidants

One of the most exciting areas of health research today is the field of antioxidant nutrients. Although antioxidants are a hot conversation topic, most people are still a little uncertain about what antioxidants really are; according to a telephone survey, more than half of Americans have heard of antioxidants, but most of those people can't actually name any antioxidant nutrients. (See "The Antioxidant Family" on page 48 for a listing of them.)

Free Radicals: The Source of the Problem

Any discussion of antioxidants must include an explanation of the oxidants that antioxidants are "against." The natural state for atoms in molecules is the possession of orbital electrons in pairs. In this state, although they can participate in reactions with other molecules, they are comparatively inert and stable. When atoms contain single, unpaired electrons, they are highly reactive, strongly seeking to pair up their electrons. They will take electrons away from other molecules less able to hold on to them. Such electron-deficient molecules are called free radicals. Of the atoms commonly found in organic molecules making up the human body, oxygen is notorious for its tendency to exist in a state with unpaired electrons. Thus free radicals of interest to us are often reactive oxygen species. When radicals are stable enough to persist for a time and migrate in tissues, they are called free radicals.

Free radicals are often highly reactive molecules that would, if left unchecked, damage the body and contribute to many diseases. Free radicals take an electron from another molecule, leaving the molecule as an

The Antioxidant Family

This chart lists antioxidants and their health benefits.

Nutrient	Benefit
Flavonoids	Prevent the formation of free radicals; protect vitamin C.
Vitamin C	Neutralizes free radicals in the watery areas of the body, such as the blood and within cells; recycles vitamin E.
Vitamin E	Protects the fatty areas of the body, such as cell membranes, from oxidation; scavenges free radicals.
Beta-carotene and other carotenoids	Scavenge singlet oxygen molecules (often resulting from sunlight exposure); prevent the oxidation of fats.
Minerals	Components of various antioxidant enzymes (e.g., superoxide dismutase, glutathione peroxidase) that mop up oxygen fragments.
Coenzyme Q_{10}	Scavenges free radicals, especially in the blood; may recycle vitamin E.
Alpha lipoic acid	Water and fat soluble substance that neutralizes free radicals all over the body; recycles vitamins C and E.

electron-deficient free radical that can take an electron from yet another molecule in a chain reaction. Some of these free radicals can react with cellular structures, causing immediate or latent damage. Antioxidants are substances that quench free radical reactions, producing harmless molecules. Antioxidants patrol the body on the lookout for free radicals. Since free radicals influence the body at such a basic level, antioxidants are an important line of defense against degenerative diseases. The human body contains a number of antioxidant molecules that can protect against the damage that reactive oxygen species and other reactive free radicals can cause, but these defenses can be overwhelmed if persistently or excessively called upon. Administration of external free radical quenchers, such as vitamin C or the antioxidants in green tea, help prevent this from happening. Cancer researchers have concluded that cancer is the consequence of the accumulation of cell damage, often caused by free radicals.

Oxygen is a paradox. Although it is absolutely essential to life, being needed in the process that converts food to energy, too much of it is damaging. In this respect, it's analogous to electricity. Electrical wires are insulated to prevent injuries from the dangerous but necessary electricity within. Similarly, antioxidants "insulate" the body from the harmful effects of oxygen. It's a good thing antioxidants are around, because free radicals just can't be avoided.

Free radicals arise from three primary sources: the body, the environment, and other free radicals.

First, the body creates some free radicals inadvertently during the complex process that derives energy from food. Exercise, illness, and certain medications can also increase the body's free radical load. On occasion, the body even deliberately creates free radicals as part of the immune system's response. Invading bacteria and other infectious microorganisms are engulfed by specialized white blood cells that use free radicals derived from oxygen to kill the potential infection-causing agents. In this isolated case, the body takes advantage of an enemy, free radicals, in order to protect itself from another enemy. Too often the reverse is true: Free radicals are the instigators of ill health.

Second, the environment is a major source of free radicals. Toxins in the environment, either natural or artificial, are often free radicals or can generate free radicals. Air pollution, toxic waste, and pesticides introduce such free radicals as nitrogen dioxide into the body. Ultraviolet radiation from the sun can produce free radicals in the skin, for example. Many people introduce free radicals into their bodies through their behaviors. Each puff of cigarette smoke contains millions of free radicals, and each swallow of alcohol leads to the production of free radicals.

Third, free radicals can be formed from other free radicals in uncontrolled chain reactions. A free radical molecule is missing a vital part of itself: one of its electrons. So, in an effort to restore the balance of paired electrons that exists in stable atoms and molecules, the free radical reacts with any nearby molecule in the body. What happens next is a deadly game of hot potato. When the original free radical "steals" an electron from another molecule, oxidation has taken place. After this oxidation, the second molecule becomes unbalanced. Since an electron has been taken from it, it is now a newly formed free radical, and it interacts with yet another molecule in pursuit of stability, and so on. These free radical chain reactions happen very quickly, in fractions of a second, but the end result can be devastating. When it is uninterrupted, the oxidation of food proceeds to the harmless generation of carbon dioxide, water, and energy, but if any of the intermediate free radicals escapes from this process, it can damage molecules in the body's cells.

Over time, free radical damage to the body leads to dozens of diseases and to premature aging. For example, free radical changes to LDL-cholesterol occur as an early stage in heart disease; damage to DNA (our genetic blueprint) caused by free radicals can instigate cancer; and proteins in the skin mangled by free radicals can appear as wrinkles. Among the most damaging of the free radicals are the superoxide ion, formed from oxygen, and the hydroxyl radical ion, formed from hydrogen peroxide. Singlet oxygen (oxygen atoms that are not bound in diatomic oxygen molecules) is another damaging free radical. Our bodies are not the only targets of free radicals. Free radical reactions are evident when a freshly cut apple begins to turn brown, oils become rancid, or rust develops on a car.

Free radical attacks on the body can be divided into four types:

1. Free radicals can oxidize the fats and proteins that compose cell membranes. This free radical damage can lead to cell membrane instability, affect the ability of the cell to access food and oxygen

and dispose of its waste products, and affect the cells' survival and reproduction.

2. Free radicals can damage the mitochondria of cells. Mitochondria are the "powerhouses" of cells where energy is actually generated. Obviously, when mitochondria are damaged, they are less effective in producing energy.

3. By deactivating enzymes and hormones, free radicals can interfere with many bodily functions, including the body's ability to grow, to repair itself, and to respond to stress.

4. When free radicals damage a cell's genetic material and alter the DNA code that governs the reproduction and function of that cell, many serious problems can develop. By some estimates, each molecule of DNA may endure as many as 10,000 free radical "hits" every day, most of which are repaired, but each of which can increase the risk of precancerous changes to the cell.[1]

Antioxidants: A Healthy Family

Antioxidants have an important ability to donate the electrons that free radicals seek, thus quenching free radicals and ending the deadly chain of free radical reactions. The spent antioxidant is then either "recycled" by yet another antioxidant to prevent its becoming a free radical itself or remains in an altered state but with a structure such that it does not damage any other molecules.

The body depends on many vitamins and minerals to act as antioxidants, and the list of compounds that can act as antioxidants is impressively long. The best free-radical protection comes from a diverse intake of antioxidants.

Plant foods are an abundant source of antioxidant nutrients, including vitamins A, C, and E, and the carotenoids. Polyphenols, the active ingredients in green tea, are especially effective antioxidants. Antioxidants serve many purposes for plants; foremost among them is protecting plants from free radicals in their environment and from free radical generators, such as ultraviolet radiation and environmental pollution. The energy in ultraviolet radiation is sufficient to turn susceptible molecules into free radicals by knocking an electron from the molecule's electron cloud. Fortunately for us, the benefits antioxidants confer to plants are transferred to us upon our ingestion of the plant or plant extract. Tea contains higher antioxidant levels than even many fruits and vegetables; drinking tea helps protect the body's cells from the damage caused by free radicals.

The body also produces antioxidant enzymes that work to convert potentially deadly free radicals into harmless substances, such as water, carbon dioxide, and ordinary oxygen. These enzymes include glutathione peroxidase, catalase, and superoxide dismutase. It was the discovery of these antioxidant enzymes in the body that convinced scientists that free radicals could cause diseases and that the body had developed ways to protect itself. These enzymes are found in every cell of the body; without them we would literally spoil. In fact, our tissues begin to rot after death in part because antioxidant enzymes have ceased to function.

Antioxidant enzyme production steps into high gear when the body is faced with increasing levels of free radicals from any source. For example, athletes have greater amounts of antioxidant enzymes than most other people because their bodies must counteract the increased amounts of free radicals produced during vigorous exercise. Under normal circumstances, the antioxidant enzymes made by the body would be sufficient to protect it from free radical damage, but modern life is anything but normal. Many things increase our free radical load, from stress to environmental toxins to a poor diet. Unfortunately, there is a limit to the body's enzyme production, and our society seems to have pushed the body to that limit. Too often, it seems, the antioxidant defenses of the body are overwhelmed, and free-radical damage accumulates and contributes to degenerative diseases. Just as a general reinforces an army with new troops, we can reinforce our body's defenses with antioxidant nutrients in our diet.

As it becomes increasingly clear that antioxidant enzymes produced in the body and the antioxidant vitamins consumed in the diet cannot completely protect all of the body's cells from oxidative damage, other antioxidants in plants, including the polyphenols found in green tea, are gaining attention. Part of the reason that a diet rich in fruits and vegetables contributes to good health is that these foods contain a great many unique antioxidants in addition to the variety of vitamins, minerals, and fiber they provide. Moreover, tea may make an even greater contribution than fruits and vegetables. In a comparison of the antioxidant activity of various vegetables (including garlic, spinach, broccoli, kale, Brussels sprouts, onions, and many others) with the antioxidant activity of green and black tea, the teas were found to have a greater ability to quench free radicals than the vegetables. Clearly, green tea is a powerful agent for fighting free radicals,[2] and it can be added to your daily antioxident arsenal in beverage or dietary supplement form.

Flavonoids: A Special Class of Antioxidants

An interesting phenomenon that can shed light on the potent antioxidant activity of polyphenols is the so-called French Paradox. As early as 1933, researchers noticed that people living in the wine-producing regions of France lived longer than the average French citizen. Later, in 1979, the British medical journal *The Lancet* published an article that built on this research, suggesting that when various countries were compared for health status, wine-drinking countries, such as France, were found to have much lower rates of heart disease. This result was particularly impressive considering all of the behaviors that would be expected to increase the risk of heart disease in the French population, such as cigarette smoking and a high-fat diet. This incongruity of a high-fat diet and high rates of smoking combined with a low risk of heart disease due to drinking red wine was dubbed the French Paradox.

What is it in red wine that exerts such powerful health protection that it can shield the body from the damage of fatty foods and cigarette smoking? Red wine is a rich source of flavonoids, a large class of antioxidant compounds that occur naturally in many plants and foods. More than four thousand flavonoids have been discovered so far in a wide variety of foods.

Three of the most powerful flavonoids in red wine are also present in green tea: catechin, epicatechin, and gallic acid. Since red wine and green tea both fight free radicals and reduce the risk of heart disease, it seems natural to assume that it is the ingredients common to both that contribute to health protection. Of late, considerable attention has been devoted by scientists to the antioxidant properties of red wine's phenolic constituent, resveratrol, as an important contributor. White wine contains much less of this antioxidant, and therefore it has fewer health benefits. Resveratrol, unfortunately, is not in green tea. However, green tea may offer even greater potential for health protection, since it not only includes the flavonoids active in red wine but also includes even more powerfully protective flavonoids that are unique to it.

When Michael G. Hertog, Ph.D., from the National Institute of Public Health and Environmental Protection in the Netherlands, assessed the intake of flavonoids in the Dutch diet, he found that "on a milligram-per-day basis, the intake of the antioxidant flavonoids still exceeded that of the antioxidants beta-carotene and vitamin E. Thus flavonoids represent an important source of antioxidants in the human diet."[3]

A well-reported 1993 study, also conducted by Dr. Hertog, showed that as intake of flavonoids increases, the risk of death from heart disease decreases. This study was based on the dietary data of approximately 800 elderly men who were followed for five years. These men were a subset of the extensive study known as the Seven Countries Study.[4]

A couple of years later, Dr. Hertog published the twenty-five-year follow-up report on the diets and mortality of more than 12,000 men involved in the Seven Countries Study. Again, there was a strong inverse relationship between flavonoid intake and death from coronary heart disease. In fact, flavonoid intake accounted for about 25 percent of the difference in heart disease risk in the groups of men.[5]

The heart is not the only part of the body to benefit from flavonoids. Another study conducted by Dutch researchers, called the Zutphen Study, found that flavonoids also protect the blood vessels. Dr. Sirving O. Kelli followed the diets of 552 middle-aged men for up to fifteen years while tracking their incidence of stroke. The men with the highest intake of flavonoids had 73 percent fewer strokes than the men with a low intake of flavonoids. Tea (black tea) was a major source of flavonoids in the diets of these men.[6]

Flavonoids, according to Professor Catherine Rice-Evans of the Free Radical Research Group at Guy's Hospital, London, perform as antioxidants through four mechanisms. These are:

- as reducing agents, disarming free radicals.
- by donating hydrogen molecules to prevent the formation of free radicals.
- by quenching singlet oxygen that would otherwise act as a free radical in the body.

- by metal chelation properties, that is, by binding with metals that could otherwise initiate the creation of free radicals. (Some metal ions, including iron and copper, promote the formation of free radicals. Chelating agents, such as certain flavonoids and EDTA, bind such ions and decrease their harmful potential.)

Professor Rice-Evans's research has determined that the flavonoids in green tea, which belong to the "catechin" family of flavonoids, have greater efficacy as antioxidants than the same quantity of vitamin C, vitamin E, or beta-carotene. However, it should be noted that flavonoids work synergistically with vitamin C and vitamin E. It is really a case of "the more the merrier" when it comes to antioxidants; it seems that there can never be too many different kinds working to neutralize free radicals.[7]

Professor Rice-Evans also determined the antioxidant activity of various green tea polyphenols with a laboratory test called the "trolox equivalent antioxidant activity measure." This test compares the free radical scavenging ability of the antioxidant in question with that of an equal amount of trolox, a water-soluble form of vitamin E. In this case the antioxidants tested included green tea polyphenols and various other flavonoids. The green tea polyphenols topped the charts. Epicatechin gallate, epigallocatechin gallate, epigallocatechin, gallic acid, epicatechin, and catechin all ranked at or near the top of the ranking for antioxidant activity.

More specifically, when Professor Rice-Evans ranked the various green tea polyphenols and adjusted for the proportion in which each is present in tea, the order from most antioxidant activity to least was found to be:

1. epigallocatechin gallate (EGCG)
2. epigallocatechin (EGC)
3. epicatechin gallate (ECG)
4. epicatechin (EC)
5. catechin (C)

These polyphenols account for 78 percent of the antioxidant potential of green tea, leaving just 22 percent contributed by as-yet-unidentified polyphenols or other substances. In terms of the polyphenols identified in this study, EGCG was the most active, accounting for 32 percent of the antioxidant potential of green tea.

The broader applicability of EGCG, EGC, and ECG over EC and C may account for their higher effectiveness. Japanese researchers discovered that the more effective green tea polyphenols are able to scavenge free radicals effectively at a wider range of pH values, whereas EC and C are limited to neutral or alkaline conditions. Fortunately, the more effective polyphenols account for the greatest proportion of those in green tea.[8]

Another antioxidant study conducted by Professor Rice-Evans assessed the ability of various green tea extracts to "spare" vitamin E from oxidation. Vitamin E is a fat-soluble antioxidant that plays an important role in preventing heart disease by neutralizing free radicals that target LDL-cholesterol. Once LDL-cholesterol is damaged by free radicals, it is more likely to contribute to atherosclerosis, the beginning stage of heart disease. Because polyphenols are water-soluble rather than fat-soluble, as vitamin E is, they cannot protect LDL-cholesterol directly; however, they may have an indirect protective effect. It has been hypothesized that green tea's polyphenols are present in the fluid surrounding LDL-cholesterol molecules, and that they quench free radicals before they even reach the LDL-cholesterol and harm it. Researchers have found that through this mechanism both EGCG and ECG delay the time until vitamin E is forced to sacrifice itself in order to prevent free radical damage to LDL-cholesterol. This may be yet another way that green tea polyphenols reduce the risk of heart disease.[9]

Green tea polyphenols prevent vitamin E from being depleted in other areas of the body. In one study, rats were fed a diet that encouraged the formation of free radicals. Under such conditions, the amount of vitamin E in the plasma of the animals' blood would be expected to decrease as the vitamin E was used to neutralize free radicals. However, when green tea extract was added to the animals' diet, it prevented the expected decrease of vitamin E, presumably because the tea extract was scavenging the free radicals and sparing the vitamin E. This effect was confirmed by the overall lower oxidative damage in rats that were fed diets supplemented with tea polyphenols.[10]

Although green tea is far superior, black tea is not without some value as an antioxidant. According to Simon Maxwell, senior lecturer at the Division of Clinical Pharmacology, Leicester Royal Infirmary, United Kingdom, black tea may account for more than half of the flavonoid intake of Western diets. Theaflavins, a group of catechins formed during the processing of black tea, are much weaker than EGCG but do show antioxidant activity in laboratory studies.[11]

Green Tea: The Polyphenol Phenom

Every kind of tea contains at least some polyphenols, but the minimal processing that green tea undergoes ensures that almost all of its poly-phenols are retained in their most reactive form in the final product, with the result that green tea has great antioxidant potential. Chi-Tang Ho, Ph.D., and colleagues from the Department of Food Science and the Center for Advanced Food Technology at Rutgers University, recently compared the free-radical-fighting ability of twelve different teas, includ-ing several varieties of green, oolong, and black teas. The results were consistent with those from other studies: Dr. Ho found that green tea had the highest yields of polyphenols—particularly for EGCG. Oolong tea was in the middle, and black tea (as a result of its auto-oxidation process) had the lowest polyphenol yield.[12]

Is the body able to absorb and use the high levels of polyphenols that green tea contains? Researchers from the Department of Nutritional Sci-ence and Dietetics at the University of Nebraska decided to answer this question by finding ten volunteers who would agree to live in their labo-ratory for two months and eat a controlled diet. During four two-week periods, the volunteers were given different beverages at each of their three meals: green tea, black tea, decaffeinated black-tea beverages, or a beverage other than tea. Their blood, urine, and feces were analyzed. Green tea resulted in the highest levels of polyphenols in the blood and waste products, followed by black tea, decaffeinated black tea, and no tea treatment. Without a doubt, green tea's polyphenols are absorbed by the body and available for use.[13]

The evidence is very clear that green tea gets your body better prepared to resist free radical attacks. When volunteers drank three cups of tea every day for two weeks, blood tests revealed that flavonoid levels jumped by 25 percent.[14] So not only does tea contain antioxidants, but these antioxidants make it into the body where they can provide protection.

Studies of the effects of tea drinking in people confirm the laboratory evidence that green tea is the most effective scavenger of free radicals. In one study, five adults each drank about two cups of green tea, while five other adults drank the same amount of black tea. The antioxidant efficacy of their blood was measured before drinking the tea, and thirty, fifty, and eighty minutes after tea ingestion. Both the green and the black teas improved the antioxidant capability of the blood, although the green tea was six times more powerful in this regard than the black tea. The increase in antioxidant function peaked within thirty minutes for the green tea drinkers and within fifty minutes for those drinking black tea. The promptness of tea's effect on blood antioxidant function suggests that the polyphenols in tea are absorbed in the upper part of the digestive tract.[15]

When it comes down to green tea extract versus free radicals, green tea comes out on top in every way. Polyphenols in green tea disarm the potentially deadly singlet oxygen. This protection from singlet oxygen is dose-dependent, meaning that the more green tea extract available to the body, the greater the protection. Not surprisingly, fresh green tea extract is a better scavenger of singlet oxygen than stale green tea extract. Green tea polyphenols are also effective in quenching hydrogen peroxide and superoxide free radicals.[16]

Green tea extract can help the body help itself, so to speak. When green tea extract is added to the drinking water of animals, their intrinsic antioxidant defense system becomes more effective. This is evidenced by an increase in antioxidant enzymes, including superoxide dismutase, glutathione reductase, glutathione peroxidase, catalase, quinone reductase, and glutathinone S-transferase. The improvement in antioxidant enzyme levels occurs throughout the body, but most notably in the lung, lower intestine, liver, and skin.[17]

The antioxidant function of green tea extract underlies almost all of the health benefits of green tea. Polyphenols prevent cardiovascular disease by shielding LDL-cholesterol from changes that promote heart disease, reduce the risk of cancer by neutralizing free radicals before genetic mutations can occur, and protect health in numerous other ways. The following chapters will cover these antioxidant-related benefits of green tea in more detail.

chapter four

Cancer Prevention in the Teapot

C ancer is one of the largest causes of death in both men and women, second only to cardiovascular disease. It claims more than six million lives each year worldwide. In fact, more than 1,500 people die every single day in the United States from cancer, while another 3,900 learn that they have this disease. Think that there's not much you can do about your risk of cancer? Think again. Diet is estimated to contribute to about one-third of preventable cancers—about the same amount as smoking. Not surprisingly, the foods that you eat tend to have the biggest impact on cancers of the digestive tract. In addition to the major risk factors of diet and smoking, differences in immune function and other lifestyle choices (exercise, for example) greatly alter your chances of developing cancer. All of these things can tip the scales in a person's favor. Green tea is one of the most promising of the cancer-fighting foods, as this chapter will show, but first let's gain a better understanding of how and why cancer develops.

The Cancer Mystery

Cancer appears to most people to be a mysterious killer that shows up unexpected and unannounced, but cancer experts do understand a lot about how cancer develops and have identified some key steps for reducing the risk of cancer, even though they are far from having a universal cancer cure. Our cells are genetically programmed by a complex set of biochemical events to stop growing when they are full-sized and have achieved their specialized character. Eventually, when they become defective, they are programmed to die and are replaced. In this way the body maintains itself. However, certain kinds of genetic damage can occur, which, if not accurately repaired, can lead to a disruption in the normal signal cells receive to stop growing. Since so many steps are normally involved in regulating cell growth, it is not uncommon for cells to require several mutations before they become fully cancerous. When this happens the cells keep on growing and dividing—crowding in on their neighbors and interfering with their proper functioning. The unrepaired damage is passed by reproduction on to progeny cells so that the defective tumor mass grows rapidly and continuously. These cells not only display continuous growth but also often fail to differentiate into functional adult cells. Some genes are more susceptible to this form of genetic damage and are often referred to as "oncogenes."

Among the means by which such transforming mutations are caused include aggressive chemicals, certain viruses, ionizing radiation, and excessive sunlight. Most DNA damage of this type is repaired, but given a sufficient number of damaging incidents the likelihood of a cancer developing is statistically more and more plausible. Early diagnosis is important so that the tumor burden does not exceed our capacity to deal with it.

Classical means of treatment involves killing the tumor mass by immune stimulation, surgery, radiation, and chemotherapy (drug treatment). It is important to remove or kill *all* of the tumor cells to prevent resumption of growth (relapse). The treatments are usually hard on patients because there are fast-growing normal cells in the body also. These include hair, immune cells, blood cells being formed in bone marrow, sperm, eggs, and the like, that are also killed along with the fast-growing tumor cells. This unfortunate circumstance leads to very unpleasant side effects associated with chemotherapy, including hair loss, susceptibility to infections, anemia, ulcers, interference with fertility, and so on. One can only conclude, therefore, that prevention is far superior to treating a cancer once it has occurred. It is in this context that antioxidants in the diet, such as those in green tea, are of great value.

Cancer is actually a group of diseases characterized by the uncontrolled growth and spread of abnormal cells. (See "The Top Ten Cancers" on page 63.) Normal, healthy cells are damaged and even destroyed when these abnormal cells invade surrounding tissues. Sometimes, cancer cells travel through the blood and lymph fluids to other parts of the body, where they initiate new cancers. This ability to form secondary cancers is called metastasis.

Cancer develops in three stages. These stages are:

1. Initiation: A substance called a mutagen or carcinogen alters a healthy cell. Cancer initiation happens quickly and frequently, but only occasionally results in an actual case of cancer.
2. Promotion: A substance called a promoter encourages the abnormal cell to multiply. The promotion stage is more lengthy, allowing the slow growth of cancer to go undetected for up to thirty years. During this time, genetic damage accumulates, making a return to normal health more and more difficult.
3. Progression: The abnormal cell growth, now called a tumor, increases in size and may spread—that is, metastasize—to other organs or tissues of the body. This stage is the deadliest.

Carcinogens are substances that trigger either the initiation or promotion stage of cancer. Carcinogens are all around us; without a watchdog system (including antioxidants) for identifying and deactivating these carcinogens, the human species would probably have died out long ago from cancer epidemics.

Although there are signs and symptoms indicating the presence of cancer, the earliest cancer symptoms—those that appear when there is the best chance of combating the disease—are often minor and vague. Consult a physician if any of the following cancer warning signs persist over several days or more:

- sudden or unexplained weight loss
- change in bowel or bladder habits
- coughing that produces bloody phlegm
- a sore that has not healed within three weeks
- a mole that itches, bleeds, or changes shape or color
- persistent hoarseness
- persistent abdominal pain

Diet, lifestyle, and the environment are responsible for initiating or promoting somewhere between 70 and 90 percent of all cancer cases. Of this, nutrition contributes between 35 and 60 percent. But keep in mind that there is rarely one single factor that results in cancer. Rather, there are many factors. (See "Cancer Factors" on page 64.)

It is estimated that two-thirds of all cancer cases could be prevented if all of the known risk factors were avoided. For instance, 90 percent of all lung cancers in men would simply not occur if no one smoked cigarettes. Avoiding other major cancer risk factors, such as excessive sun exposure, alcohol, asbestos, pesticides, and some food additives, could also reduce the incidence of cancer.

Some substances in food are major contributors to cancer, including some that occur naturally and others that are added in processing. For example, food additives called nitrites, found in processed meats such as bacon and bologna, are converted in the body to potent carcinogens called nitrosamines. Other dietary mutagens include aflatoxin (a natural substance produced by a mold that forms on improperly stored peanuts); heavy metals, such as lead; polychlorinated biphenyls (PCBs); and pesticides, such as malathion and DDT. Alcohol does not initiate cancer, but it promotes the growth of a pre-existing abnormal cell. Examples of other suspected dietary promoters are saccharin, excess dietary fat, and excessive use of coffee or caffeine. It is estimated by cancer researchers that the incidence of gastric carcinoma in the United States has decreased by three-fourths in the last fifty years simply by improving means of preserving meat and reduced use of nitrites.

Anti-Cancer Dietary Advice

Although a person's diet is a source of carcinogens, the good news is that the diet also contains many substances that prevent the development or progression of cancer. The National Cancer Institute has developed a set of dietary guidelines for minimizing the risk of developing cancer. These guidelines advise people to lower their fat intake, increase fiber intake, choose plentiful amounts of fruits and vegetables, maintain an ideal body weight, use alcohol in moderation, and avoid certain processed foods.

The Top Ten Cancers*

The following are the ten most common types of cancer for men and women, ranked in order from one to ten.

For Men	For Women
1. Prostate	1. Breast
2. Lung	2. Lung
3. Colon and Rectum	3. Colon and Rectum
4. Bladder	4. Uterus
5. Lymphoma	5. Lymphoma
6. Skin	6. Skin
7. Kidney	7. Thyroid
8. Leukemia	8. Ovary
9. Oral	9. Kidney
10. Pancreas	10. Leukemia

* 2007 estimates from the American Cancer Society.

Limit Fat Intake to 30 Percent of Calories or Less

Research studies of animals and humans show that a high-fat diet increases the risk of many cancers, including colon and prostate cancer. Conversely, a low-fat diet has been shown to reduce the risk of many cancers. An additional benefit of a low-fat diet is the fact that it helps most people maintain a healthy weight. Besides total fat intake, the type of fat in the diet appears to affect cancer risk. There are many different types of dietary fat; some have tumor-promoting properties, and others have tumor-inhibiting properties.

Saturated fat has the strongest link to colon and prostate cancer. Some research shows polyunsaturated fat to have a moderately significant relationship to cancer. Unsaturated fatty acids and the trans-fatty acids formed in the processing of foods have also been implicated in cancer. However, diets high in the omega-3 fatty acids found in fish oils have been show to reduce the growth of cancerous tumor cells. Research indicates that supplementing a person's diet with omega-3 fatty acids significantly reduces the risk of colon cancer.

Consume 20 to 30 Grams of Fiber Per Day

A diet high in fiber helps prevent cancer in several ways. First, fiber-rich foods are generally low in fat and calories and are loaded with other

Cancer Factors

The following factors contribute to the development of cancer:

- **Pro-carcinogens:** initially harmless substances that may be altered in the body to induce cancer.

Examples: The polycyclic aromatic hydrocarbons (PAHs) that are present in condensed smoke from cigarettes, automobile emissions, grilled foods, fireplace residues, and the like are examples. Largely inert by themselves, liver enzymes can attack these substances with reactive oxygen species to produce carcinogens that react with DNA unless intercepted and deactivated. Certain nitrogen-containing molecules produced by cooking, especially grilling red meats or in Cajun-style blackening of meats, serve as pro-carcinogens.

- **Carcinogens:** substances that increase the risk of cancer.

Examples: Some chemicals are sufficiently reactive that they can attack DNA without requiring metabolic activation. Examples are alkylating agents, such as dimethyl sulfate and diazomethane, encountered primarily in industrial research laboratories. Ultraviolet rays from sunlight or tanning parlors are another example.

- **Initiators:** substances that, under certain conditions, produce a cancerous cell.

Examples: Attack of DNA by carcinogens or the metabolites of pro-carcinogens can result in initiation.

- **Promoters:** substances that cause a cell that is "primed" for cancer to become cancerous.

Examples: Alcohol, teleocidin (a mold product), and croton oil, which contains 12-0-tetradecanoylphorbol-13-acetate, are examples of promoters. Croton oil was used as a strong laxative until about a generation ago. Dioxins and asbestos also fit in this category.

- **Co-carcinogens:** substances that contribute to tumor growth.

Examples: An example of this is the enzyme P-450. More examples are: hydrogen peroxide, estrogens (suspected), sulfur dioxide, ferric oxide and alcohol.

Aligned against those factors are the **anti-carcinogens**, substances that inhibit carcinogens.

Examples: Certain sulfur-containing molecules found in cruciferous vegetables (Brussels sprouts, broccoli, etc.) detoxify directly by acting as alkylating agents, and certain antioxidants, such as epigallocatechin gallate from green tea and resveratrol from red wine and grape juice, inhibit the oxidative metabolism of pro-carcinogens to carcinogens.

valuable nutrients. Second, fiber has been shown to bind with cancer-causing substances in the colon, shuttling them harmlessly out of the body. (Note that daily fiber intake should not exceed 35 grams.)

Eat a Variety of Vegetables and Fruits Daily

Fruits and green, leafy vegetables are a veritable treasure trove of important vitamins, minerals, and, particularly, antioxidants. They are high in fiber, low in fat, and supply vitamin-like compounds called phytonutri-ents. Green tea falls into this category of recommendations.

Avoid Obesity

Research shows that a person 40 percent or more above his or her ideal weight has a 33 percent greater risk of developing cancer than a person who is not overweight. Conversely, weight reduction can reduce the risk of cancer in obese people.

Consume Alcoholic Beverages in Moderation, If at All

In addition to causing cirrhosis, which can lead to liver cancer, alcohol abuse increases the risk for cancers of the oral cavity, larynx, and esoph-agus. This risk is intensified in alcohol abusers who also smoke.

Minimize Consumption of Salt-Cured, Salt-Pickled, or Smoked Foods

Nitrates and nitrites, common preservatives used in the processing of meats, can form nitrosamines, which in turn can cause cancer. The smoking of foods also can increase the risk of cancer. Cooking fatty cuts of meat over an open fire or barbecue can result in the formation of car-cinogens or pro-carcinogenic substances in the meat.

Green Tea's Anti-Cancer Mechanisms

Many years ago, scientists dismissed green tea's reputation as a health-enhancing beverage as folklore, even though it can be traced back thou-sands of years. This dismissal changed to respect when epidemiologists, scientists who study the risk of disease and death among groups of people over time, discovered that Asians rank at the top in worldwide compari-sons of disease and health. In other words, Asians have a lower risk of getting, or dying from, many diseases that plague most Western coun-tries. When researchers took a closer look at the statistics to determine the relative importance of factors that could affect health, such as access to medical care, smoking, genetic differences, and pollution, they concluded that there must be something in the diet to account for Asian health.

Even within Asian countries, diet seems to affect disease rates from region to region. Take, for example, the Shizuoka Prefecture of Japan. This area of Japan has a much lower death rate from cancer for both men and women than does the country as a whole, according to vital statistics gathered by the Japanese Ministry of Health and Welfare. Intrigued by this phenomenon, epidemiologists decided to delve deeper. They discovered that green tea was a staple product in the tea-producing Shizuoka region; people living in this area drank more cups of green tea than the average Japanese. It seemed logical, these scientists suggested, that drinking green tea contributed to the surprisingly lower cancer rates, but this statistical relationship was not enough to prove the link. Scientists began dozens of experiments to determine whether their theory was true. Does green tea reduce the risk of cancer? Let's see what they found out.

Investigations into the effects of green tea included laboratory experiments, experiments on animals, experiments on humans consuming various ordinary diets, and statistical studies of human populations. One of the most convincing studies was undertaken not in Asia but in Iowa. Epidemiologists from the University of Minnesota sent a questionnaire to 35,369 middle-aged Iowa women asking questions about their health status, lifestyle, and diet (including their average daily tea intake). The epidemiologists tracked the health status of these women for the next eight years, noting how many developed cancer. During that time, 2,936 women were diagnosed with cancer.[1]

Overall, about 40 percent of these Iowa women drank tea (green, black, or oolong) at least once a week, and almost 20 percent drank tea every day, with half of the group drinking two or more cups daily. The women who drank the most tea were found to have a 10 percent lower incidence of cancers of any type compared with the women as a whole. Specifically, frequent tea drinkers had almost 70 percent fewer cancers of the digestive tract and 40 percent fewer urinary tract cancer cases compared with women who rarely or never drank tea. It's hard to question a study this thorough and results this strong. Clearly, tea, in some way, lessens the risk of cancer.

The concept of chemoprevention may help explain how green tea reduces cancer risks. Cancer chemoprevention is a means of controlling cancer, even in the face of cancer-causing agents, by increasing a person's exposure to certain cancer-fighting compounds. These chemopreventive compounds are technically called anti-carcinogens; ideally, they should be nontoxic as well, Chemoprevention is different from cancer treatment, since chemoprevention's goal is to lower the incidence of cancer rather than to treat existing cancers. After they have been identified in foods, these chemopreventive agents are generally extracted so that they can be administered more conveniently and at a standardized dosage.

An advantage of green tea extract and other nutrients over pharmaceutical drugs in cancer therapy is that the nutrients are generally less potent and can be used safely over a much wider range of dosages, so they are safer to use. Pharmaceutical drugs are safe and effective only within a narrow range of dosage. In large doses they become toxic and can do more harm than good, so doses must be carefully established and prescribed. For nutritional supplements, the safety range is dramatically larger, making them safer to use. Even in the case of nutritional supplements, however, safe dosage limits should not be exceeded, so manufacturers often print recommended daily intake levels on the labels, and these should not be exceeded.

As an alternative to recommending that cancer-conscious individuals drink multiple cups of green tea daily, some agriculturists are devising ways of upping the level of active ingredients in tea plants, particularly the catechin EGCG. This would result in higher EGCG levels in every cup. The focus on EGCG levels is appropriate, since a study reported in the journal *Anti-Cancer Drugs* determined that "EGCG was the most potent of the seven green tea components [investigated in the study] against three out of the four cell lines" tested for cancer prevention. According to research conducted by John H. Weisburger from the American Health Foundation, future selective breeding of tea plants may boost the anti-cancer activity of tea further. Whether this effort will produce cups of tea that would be as delicious, healthful, and safe as the natural plants remains to be seen. Meanwhile, supplements of green-tea extracts in tablet and capsule form that are standardized for high levels of EGCG would seem to achieve this increase indirectly.[2]

"Due to the many biological activities of tea polyphenols, more than one mechanism could be important in the inhibition of carcinogenesis by tea," Theresa J. Smith from Rutgers University reminds us. Dr. Smith details a list of ways green tea extract undermines cancer, including preventing DNA strand breaks, inhibiting cell proliferation, decreasing the contact of carcinogens with cells, blocking cancer initiation, and slowing cancer progression.[3] Let's take a closer look at each of these.

Preventing DNA Strand Breaks

As we saw in the previous chapter, free radicals are the underlying instigators of a number of degenerative diseases afflicting man, and cancer is one of them. Of the various types of cellular damage that can be caused by free radicals, damage to DNA (our genetic blueprint) is potentially the most dangerous to the whole animal. When DNA replicates itself, unrepaired damage caused by free radicals is preserved through inappropriate base substitutions and often even magnified in the succeeding DNA generations. Cancer is now generally considered a consequence of the failure of cells to undergo normally regulated growth.

Cancer researchers have concluded that an initial DNA injury develops into active cancer through the accumulation over time of specific DNA defects in certain target cells. The instigating free radical "hit" may have occurred many years before the cancer transformation is complete and an actual disease state is discernible. This long interval of latency makes it difficult for scientists to establish, without a doubt, the particular cause-and-effect relationships for cancer; however, you can use this long period to your advantage by adding to your diet chemopreventive agents that will thwart the progress of cancer.

According to free radical experts, each molecule of DNA in our bodies can receive thousands of free radical "hits" each day and continue unaffected by the insult. This resilience arises from the fact that the body is continually restoring and repairing itself, but the body is not invincible. If a free radical-damaged DNA sequence is not excised and repaired before a cell divides, the damage becomes permanent through alterations in the DNA structure, and potentially cancerous. The body may fail to correct a particular free radical hit if antioxidant levels are low.

Blocking Cancer Initiation

The antioxidant capabilities of green tea are the primary mechanism by which green tea prevents the initiation of cancer. Green tea's catechins supplement the body's levels of antioxidants, which neutralize free radicals before they even have a chance to interact with DNA. In addition, green tea boosts the body's levels of antioxidant enzymes. Researchers at the Case Western Reserve University in Cleveland, Ohio, suggest that increased activities of the glutathione peroxidase, catalase, and quinone reductase enzymes in numerous organ systems of animals, including the skin, bowel, liver, and lung, is "one of the possible mechanisms of cancer chemopreventive effects associated with green tea."[4]

Another anti-cancer benefit of green tea is its ability to block the formation of carcinogenic nitrosamines from the nitrites and nitrates in processed meats that would otherwise increase the risk of stomach cancer. As little as three to five grams of tea daily, Dr. Smith estimates, would be sufficient to block nitrosamine formation, which would significantly lower the incidence of stomach cancer. Other researchers from China confirm that green tea inhibits the transformation of nitrosamines. This conclusion was reached after testing 145 different samples of green, oolong, and black tea. Incidentally, drinking tea before a meal that contained nitrites and nitrates was more effective than drinking tea after the meal, researchers found. It seems that the polyphenols in the tea react with the nitrosamine compounds in order to reduce their carcinogenic activity or prevent their formations.[5]

Green tea extract also offers the promise of preventing cancer by inhibiting the activation of carcinogens. A study published in the journal *Food & Chemical Toxicology* found that rats administered the equivalent of a human dose of green tea had a lower risk of cancer because "the anticarcinogenic effect of green tea facilitated the metabolism of chemical carcinogens into inactive, readily excretable products."[6]

Mutagens are a broad range of compounds that cause genetic mutations; these mutations often instigate the initiation stage of cancer. Several studies conducted in cells grown in laboratory dishes (called *in vitro* studies) revealed that green tea polyphenols "decrease the mutagenicity of several mutagens and carcinogens." Other studies identified the primary antimutagenic compound in green tea specifically as EGCG. Other anti-mutagenic compounds in green tea include caffeine and vitamin C.[7]

Antimutagenic compounds can be further categorized according to their modes of action. Experts suggest that *desmutagens* inactivate mutagens through chemical or enzymatic interactions with them, thereby preventing the alteration of genes. Meanwhile, *bioantimutagens* lessen the damage after genes have been attacked by mutagens by helping the gene repair itself or by lessening the impact the mutated gene has on other parts of the cell. According to Dr. Yu F. Sasaki from the University of Shizuoka in Japan, "both desmutagenic and bioantimutagenic activity of green tea catechins have been reported."[8]

Inhibiting Cell Proliferation and Slowing Cancer Progression

One of the common scientific analyses used to assess the success of antimutagenic compounds involves the fruit fly. The larvae of this fly are grown in a medium containing known mutagens, with a portion of the larvae also exposed to potential antimutagenic compounds. The appearance of spots on the wings of the adult flies serves as an indication of the severity of mutations. When researchers from the Okayama University in Japan added EGCG extracted from green tea to the larvae's growth medium, the wing spot formations were dramatically inhibited, and the more EGCG given to the developing larvae, the stronger the inhibitory effect. The researchers suspect that the green tea extract blocked mutagens from entering the cells of the insects. The researchers hypothesize that a similar effect occurs in humans.[9]

The cells of the body must be able to communicate with one another so as to coordinate their growth and metabolism. The better the cells can communicate, the stronger are their defenses against cancer, since the cells can monitor one another for changes that are characteristic of cancer development. On the other hand, when communication is shut down, the uncontrolled growth of abnormal and cancerous cells is more likely. This communication between cells transpires through chemical hormones via membrane-bound protein receptors. Other receptors in the cell cytosol transmit these messages toward the nucleus, where yet more receptors cause or prevent the synthesis of cellular materials. The degree of synthetic activity is important to keep cell growth in tissues in harmony. Derangements in this cellular signaling system can lead to cell death or immortalization, as in cancer. Another means of cellular communication is through gap junctions, protein tubes piercing the cell membranes of adjoining cells and so permitting cytoplasmic contact between them. Green tea polyphenols protect this delicately balanced communication system between cells from free radical damage, which is yet another way that green tea may help prevent cancer.[10] Ongoing research continues to support a role of green tea in positively affecting cell signaling pathways that prevent the transformation of healthy cells to cancerous cells.[11]

Cancerous tumors are made up of undifferentiated cells. Differentiation is the process that tells a developing cell to become a heart cell, a nerve cell, and so on. Without differentiation, a cell does not have a clearly defined "job description," and uncontrolled cancerous growth can result. The polyphenols in green tea help prevent cancer by diminishing the cell damage that would otherwise inhibit the differentiation of developing cells into normal, healthy cells.

Decreasing the Contact of Carcinogens with Cells

An enzyme called ornithine decarboxylase (ODC) is the "rate-limiting enzyme" in cancer growth. All cells need the product of ODC in order to initiate cell division. Without ODC, cancerous cells cannot proliferate and normal cells cannot be transformed into cancerous cells; when ODC is no longer available, the tumor cannot continue to grow. Consequently, agents that block induction of ODC can prevent the growth of tumors. A study conducted at the Chinese Academy of Preventive Medicine reports that when mice prone to developing skin cancer are given EGCG, the effects of ODC are significantly lessened. Furthermore, the blocking of ODC occurs in a dose-dependent manner; that is, higher concentrations of green tea polyphenols result in a greater inhibition of the ODC enzyme.[12]

Carcinogens are potentially dangerous by themselves. When pro-carcinogens are "activated" by enzymes in the body they can become particularly nasty. The cytochrome P450 enzymes in the liver have the potential to activate pro-carcinogens to highly reactive species, which can then attack DNA and other components of the body's cells. Fortunately, many chemopreventive compounds block the P450-related activation of pro-carcinogens. Not surprisingly, green tea extract is among these chemopreventive agents, and EGCG is one of the most powerful of the polyphenols with this function.[13]

Additional Cancer Fighting Methods

Recently, it has been discovered that EGCG in tea leads some tumor cells to essentially commit suicide, a process scientists call "apoptosis." Programmed cell death is another name for apoptosis, and it is an orderly process that is an important part of the life cycle. Apoptosis is increasingly believed to be a very important way that green tea fights cancer development.[14] During the development and spread of cancer, not enough cells are engaged in apoptosis, so the increase in new cell numbers progressively exceeds the number of cells that are dying. In addition, EGCG blocks a process called angiogenesis, which is the process of forming new blood vessels. This is something that growing tumors need to support their harmful growth and spread. Yet another way that green tea fights cancer is by reducing the chances that an existing tumor will spread (metastasis) to additional locations in the body.

Perhaps the researchers at the National Cancer Center Research Institute in Tokyo, Japan, provide the best overall summation regarding the cancer-preventing abilities of green tea extract: "We suggest drinking green tea may be one of the most practical methods of cancer prevention available at the present."[15] In the next chapter, we'll investigate how green tea and polyphenols successfully prevent cancers that strike specific organs and tissues of the body, as well as how green tea supports the body during chemotherapy and radiation cancer therapy.

chapter five

Tea's Effect on Cancers and Side Effects of Cancer Treatments

A lthough fatal cases of cancer have decreased slightly, cancer is poised to become this country's top killer—mostly because cancer fatalities are not decreasing as rapidly as heart-disease fatalities. As we've seen, green tea works through several mechanisms to reduce the overall risk of cancer; in addition, polyphenols have been shown to prevent cancers that may develop in specific organs or tissues of the body. The following sections detail the promising research that links green tea polyphenols to the prevention of individual cancers. Moreover, green tea appears to have very special qualities that ease the adverse effects of conventional cancer treatments, such as radiation and chemotherapy.

Skin Cancer

More than 2 million new cases of skin cancer are diagnosed every year, but, fortunately, the majority of these are basal cell cancer and squamous cell cancers, which are highly curable if caught in time. Only 62,000 of the annual cases are the deadly melanoma cancer that accounts for three-quarters of the fatal cases of skin cancer. The number one risk factor for skin cancer is exposure to ultraviolet (UV) radiation from the sun. Skin cancer is more common in people with fair skin that burns or freckles easily; thus Caucasians are forty times more likely to develop skin cancer than are blacks. The warning signs of skin cancer include a mole that changes in any way or other skin changes. The initiating exposure can take place long before detectable cancer develops. The skin changes can be remembered conveniently as the ABCDs:

A   Asymmetry or irregular growth
B   Borders irregular
C   Color variations within the growth
D   Diameter exceeding 6 millimeters

Laboratory experiments using cells grown in petri dishes and experiments performed under standardized conditions with laboratory animals indicate that green tea extract taken orally or applied directly to the skin offers significant protection against skin cancer caused by UV radiation or external exposure to cancer-causing chemicals.

The preeminent researcher in the field of chemoprevention of skin cancer is Santosh K. Katiyar, Ph.D., from the Department of Dermatology at the Case Western Reserve University in Cleveland, Ohio. He has designed and completed several studies investigating green tea's ability to prevent skin cancer in the mouse skin cancer model. Dr. Katiyar's research series has demonstrated that green tea protects against cancers caused by UV radiation, and that a green tea cream applied prior to exposure to a carcinogen is highly effective in protecting the skin against cancerous changes. Mice in a group that was treated with a green tea cream developed fewer and smaller tumors than did mice that were not administered the cream. Dr. Katiyar also found that green tea extract lessens swelling of the skin and uncontrolled growth of skin cells in mice. Green tea extract shows the most protective effect when it is administered before cancer develops, but significant protective effects were noticeable throughout all cancer stages. The progression of skin cancer is lessened by topically applied green tea. As a whole, Dr. Katiyar's body of research shows that green tea extract has a protective effect in all three stages of cancer: initiation, promotion, and progression. Studies by other researchers even show that green tea extract inhibits development of melanoma, the most deadly form of skin cancer.[1]

Research in humans follows right in line with the animal models. Drinking tea lowers the risk of squamous cell carcinoma. Applying green tea polyphenols to the skin before UV exposure blocks DNA damage.

And it is interesting to note that green tea in general and EGCG in isolation have both been documented for averting photoaging of the skin.[2]

Esophageal Cancer

Green tea has a less clear-cut role in esophageal cancer than in cancers of other sites. Some preliminary studies showed that green tea protected against esophageal cancer, while other studies suggested an alarming *increased* risk of cancer of the esophagus in those drinking green tea. A closer examination of the research offers a plausible explanation of the conflicting studies: differences in beverage temperature. Epidemiological studies of human populations show that people who drink tea at a normal, hot temperature (95°F to 115°F) do not have a higher risk of cancer; however, when tea is consumed at extremely hot temperatures (above 130°F), it can scald the delicate lining of the esophagus, making the risk of cancer as much as three times greater.[3] Thus the action responsible for developing cancer is more likely to be the excessive heat than the tea. It would be interesting to see whether the ingestion of hot water instead of hot tea would produce similar findings. This risk can be eliminated by taking green tea in supplement form.

Cancer researchers at the Chinese Academy of Preventive Medicine in Beijing, China, presented the results of their studies of the preventive effect of tea polyphenols on esophageal cancer in rats to the 1991 First International Symposium on the Physiological and Pharmacological Effects of *Camellia sinensis* (Tea). A group of rats was exposed to cancer-promoting chemicals that would normally result in esophageal tumors in 95 percent of the animals. Some of the rats were also given tea extracts from green, black, and oolong tea; only 5 to 19 percent of rats given tea extracts developed cancers of the esophagus. Additionally, the tumors in the tea-treated animals that did develop cancer were smaller in size and fewer in number than the tumors developed by the rats not given tea extracts. Other indications of poor esophageal health, such as precancerous lesions and abnormal skin growth, were also less frequent in the rats treated with tea extract.[4]

In another animal study, this one conducted at Rutgers University in New Jersey, green tea extract reduced the incidence of esophageal tumors by 50 percent when it was given after exposure to cancer-promoting chemicals and by 70 percent when it was present in the diet before and during exposure.[5]

Animal studies are suggestive, but evidence from studies of human populations would be more clearly pertinent. Researchers from the National Cancer Institute in the United States and the Shanghai Cancer Institute in China teamed up in 1994 to use epidemiological methods to investigate the effects of green tea in a human population. A cancer registry in China identified 902 esophageal cancer patients, and another 1,552 cancer-free men and women were included in the study as controls. All of these men and women were interviewed to gather information about diet, medical history, smoking status, alcohol use, tea drinking habits, family history of cancer, occupation, physical activity, and reproductive history. Statistical analysis of the data showed that alcohol users and cigarette smokers have "risk reductions [for developing esophageal cancer] of about 20% among male and 50% among female drinkers of green tea. For nonsmokers and nonalcohol drinkers . . . risks were reduced by 57% for men and 60% for women by green tea drinking." This study could be promising news for the approximately 15,000 Americans diagnosed with esophageal cancer every year in the United States.[6]

Oral Cancer

Oral cancer (sometimes called mouth cancer) generally involves the lips, tongue, or cheek lining. Tobacco use (either smoking or chewing tobacco) is implicated in up to 80 percent of oral cancer cases. Heavy alcohol use is another risk factor. When people with leukoplakia (precancerous lesions) in the mucus lining of their mouths were treated with a tea product for six months, lesions had at least a partial regression in 38 percent of the group (compared with 10 percent of those who were treated with a placebo). Animal model research follows in line with this human study, showing that oral cancers are either less likely to develop or tumors are smaller when animals drink tea.[7]

Gastrointestinal Tract Cancer

For someone who will develop cancer this year, there is a one in five chance that it will be in the digestive system, such as the colon/rectum or stomach. Drinking tea puts this beverage in direct contact with the gastrointestinal tract, which is why scientists have kept their eye on potential benefits from green tea for various cancers of the digestive system. Although there are several promising studies (which will be detailed in this section), it should also be noted that there is research that failed to document beneficial effects of green tea for digestive cancers. Even so, there continue to be glimmers of hope in the research in favor of green tea in the treatment of stomach cancer, such as a study based on 18,000 men in Shanghai that showed a significant inverse relationship between tea polyphenol levels (as measured in urine) and risk of gastric cancer.[8]

The Japanese region of Shizuoka is noted for an unexpectedly low overall incidence of cancer and an especially low incidence of stomach cancer. The fact that the people of this region are also known to drink more than an average amount of green tea sparked several epidemiological research studies into the possibility of a causal relationship between green tea and reduced incidence of stomach cancer. A Japanese study that compared the tea-drinking habits of 139 patients with stomach cancer and 2,852 people without stomach cancer revealed that people who drank large quantities of green tea (ten or more cups daily) had a much lower risk of developing cancer of the stomach than those who did not. The results of another case-control study, in which the dietary habits of a group of people with cancer are compared with the dietary habits of a similar group of people who do not have the disease, this one conducted in China and involving 1,422 individuals, indicated that the risk of developing cancer of the stomach is 29 percent lower for green tea drinkers than for those who don't drink green tea. The researchers who conducted this study suggested that green tea may disrupt the intermediate and late stages in the development of stomach cancer. Furthermore, other research has shown that green tea has an inhibitory effect on cancers that may develop in the cardia and distal areas of the stomach. Researchers from the British Columbia Cancer Research Center in Canada concluded that "the simultaneous intake of teas with food products that . . . [increase the risk of stomach cancer] . . . of human subjects should exert a protective, beneficial effect.[9]

Farther along the digestive tract, just past the stomach, lies the small intestine. In this organ, too, green tea extract exerts a protective effect, according to results from laboratory experiments on animals. Scientists from the Food Research Laboratories, located in the Shizuoka area of Japan now famous for reduced risks of cancer, found that the incidence of small intestine cancer in rats exposed to carcinogens declined significantly if they were also exposed to green tea extract. Other Japanese researchers agree with this finding. In studies of cancer in mice, animals fed a diet supplemented with EGCG developed half as many tumors of the small intestine as did animals without supplements. Cancers of the large intestine are also less common when animals are fed polyphenols from green tea, say researchers from Henan Medical University in China.[10]

The final segment of the digestive tract is comprised of the colon and rectum. Cancer of the colon or rectum is the third most common cause of cancer deaths in the United States, and more than 153,000 new cases are diagnosed every year. Chemoprevention of colon and rectum cancer is particularly important for two reasons. First, the rate of mortality from colon cancer has not changed substantially over the past several decades, despite intensive efforts at treatment, suggesting that prevention is at present a better strategy than chemotherapy for controlling this disease. Second, the fact that colon cancer can be caused or exacerbated by environmental factors suggests that it might be prevented or inhibited by altering these environmental factors, specifically, by adding to the diet foods that contain cancer-preventing agents. Colon cancer rates in Asian countries are much lower than colon cancer rates in the United States and Europe. Since many people in Asia drink plenty of green tea, could this be one of the sources of the difference?

In terms of gastrointestinal health, the benefits from drinking tea are cumulative (meaning they add up) in terms of how long you have been drinking tea and how many cups you drink each day. For example, in one study with women who drank about 2.5 cups of tea daily, they had a 60 percent risk reduction for rectal cancer, compared to women drinking less than 1.2 cups daily. Another study of tea drinkers found a 42 percent lower risk of colon cancer (again, compared to non–tea drinkers), and if the men in this study drank more than 1.5 cups of tea each day, they had a 70 percent lower risk of colon cancer.[11]

The research data for assessing green tea's potential as a chemopreventive agent against colon and rectum cancer would benefit from more human studies, but the data available from animal studies are promising.

According to a study conducted at the University of Hawaii, green tea extracts administered to rats exposed to cancer-promoting substances protected the rats' DNA against alteration. More specifically, green tea extract inhibits colon cancer progression, as indicated by a lower incidence of crypt cells in the colon, which are indications of cancer progression. Additional experiments on animals have confirmed this finding. Green tea extract protects the mucus lining of the colon from free radical damage and, even at very low doses, prevents the formation of colon tumors. In one study, researchers found only half as many tumors in the colons of animals that had been given green tea polyphenols. Of the few human studies, one—an epidemiological study—revealed that older Japanese men who drink greater amounts of green tea tend to have decreased risk of developing adenomatous polyps (which can progress to colon cancer).[12]

And in another human trial, when researchers followed more than 34,000 postmenopausal women for a dozen years, they found that the women who consumed the highest level of catechins had a 45 percent drop in rectal cancer cases. Furthermore, another large study found an inverse relationship between drinking green tea and the risk of colon and rectal cancers. In this study, men who drank 4.5 cups of tea daily had an 18 percent reduction in risk of colon cancer and a 28 percent lowering of rectal cancer risk. For women, drinking three cups daily dropped colon and rectal cancer risk by 33 percent and 43 percent respectively.[13]

Lung Cancer

Lung cancer is a leading cause of mortality in men and women. Most cases of lung cancer can be traced back to exposure to carcinogens, mostly from cigarette smoking, but also from exposure to asbestos, radiation, and radon. Green tea extract is a very promising chemopreventive agent against lung cancer, since many experiments on laboratory animals indicate that it ameliorates the effects of chemical carcinogens. In a study that focused on lung cancer in particular, researchers at the Department of Veterans Affairs Medical Center in Cleveland, Ohio found that mice exposed to carcinogens developed 55 percent fewer lung tumors if they were given polyphenols extracted from green tea. Japanese researchers discovered that metastasis of lung tumors was significantly reduced when mice were given a green tea infusion to drink. In other research, 80 percent of a control group of mice developed cancerous and precancerous lesions, while only 14 percent of the mice in a group that drank green tea developed such lesions.[14]

In studies of human populations, the results have not been as clear-cut. A cohort study of men in London suggested that drinking black tea increased, rather than minimized, the risk of lung cancer. A handful of other studies of human populations failed to find any relationship—positive or negative—between tea consumption and lung cancer. In order to reconcile these equivocal findings, researchers from the Nagoya University School of Medicine in Japan analyzed data gathered in the Okinawa prefecture, an area of Japan with the highest rate of mortality from lung cancer of all the forty-seven Japanese prefectures. In Okinawa in 1992, the rate was 38.2 deaths from lung cancer per 100,000 men and 10.2 per 100,000 women. In comparison, the rates of mortality from lung cancer for all of Japan in that year were 30.3 for men and 7.9 for women.

The people in this area of Japan drink what they call "Okinawan" tea, which is similar to green tea, although it is very slightly auto-oxidated (even less so than oolong tea). Chemical analyses of the polyphenol content of Okinawan tea are, unfortunately, not available; however, the researchers who conducted the Okinawa study believe that, since it is very similar to green tea, it also has high levels of EGCG. The statistics compiled in this study were based on 333 men and women diagnosed with primary lung cancer and 666 cancer-free individuals matched by age and sex. The degree of lung cancer protection derived from drinking Okinawan tea was greater for women than men. Drinking one to nine cups of tea daily lowered the risk of developing lung cancer by 23 percent in the females. Women who drank ten or more cups daily had their risk of lung cancer slashed an amazing 62 percent. For the men, drinking one to nine cups of tea daily reduced cancer risk by 15 percent, and drinking ten or more cups daily cut cancer risk by 43 percent. "In short," said the researchers, "our study found that the greater the intake of Okinawan tea, the smaller the lung cancer risk, and suggested an inhibitory effect of tea consumption on the development of lung cancer in humans."[15]

Doctors agree that the incidence of lung cancer would plummet if people would stop smoking, since smoking is linked to 90 percent of all lung cancer cases. Numerous carcinogens are present in cigarette smoke.

One in particular is highly correlated to the development of lung cancer; it is a nitrosamine called NNK that is produced by processing or burning tobacco. Cancer researchers have concluded that the cytochrome P450 enzymes in the liver "potentiate" NNK by oxidizing it, making it an activated carcinogen. The fact that lung cancer mortality rates are lower in Japan than in the United States, even though Japanese men are twice as likely to smoke as American men, is consistent with the view that lifestyle factors or diet inhibit the activation of tobacco carcinogens.

Experiments on animals indicate that the polyphenols in green tea ameliorate the damage caused by NNK. When mice are treated with NNK they develop an average of 22.5 lung tumors per mouse, scientists from the American Health Foundation report. But when EGCG is added to their water, only 16.1 tumors develop. Based on the amounts of EGCG given to these animals, it seems that as small a dose of EGCG as that found in a daily cup of green tea would lessen the impact of NNK in humans. Other animal research indicates that EGCG blocks about 50 percent of the harmful effects of NNK and may accomplish the blockage by interacting with the P450 enzyme system.[16]

The data gathered from studies of human smoking populations falls in line with the results from animal studies. Blood markers of tobacco-related carcinogens were measured in fifty-two healthy men aged twenty to fifty-two, as were their rates of consumption of green tea. The men who regularly drank green tea had blood profiles similar to that of a nonsmoker, while the men who did not drink green tea showed unhealthy levels of tobacco-derived carcinogens in their blood. Although not smoking is the obvious first choice for health, regular consumption of green tea may offer those who do smoke some protection from the carcinogens that are present in tobacco smoke.[17]

Prostate Cancer

Cancer of the prostate is a common cancer in American men; approximately 27,000 Americans die of it each year. The evidence for green tea's role in the prevention or slowed progression of prostate cancer is generally positive, based on laboratory and animal studies.[18] Japan tells quite a different story; they have the lowest rate of prostate cancer in the world. (The prostate is a male gland located under the bladder.) When people emigrate from a country with a low incidence of cancer to one with a high incidence, their cancer risk typically rises to match that of their new home. Researchers wondered whether Japanese men would continue to enjoy a low level of cancer risk even if they moved to a high-risk country.

Richard K. Severson, the lead researcher for the Japan-Hawaii Cancer Study, investigated this question by interviewing about eight thousand Japanese men living in Hawaii and charting cases of prostate cancer for as long as twenty-one years. During that period, 174 men developed prostate cancer. Only one-tenth of this number of men would have been expected to develop prostate cancer if they had been living in Japan. Clearly, environment, lifestyle, and diet played key roles in raising the risk of prostate cancer.[19]

It is likely that as they acclimatized themselves to life in their new country, the Japanese men began to consume more American-style meals. This dietary change would account for the rising rate of cases of prostate cancer. However, by retaining some of the traditional elements of their diets, the men preserved some of their enviably low risk of prostate cancer. Despite their increased risk of cancer relative to men in Japan, they were still less likely to develop the disease than most American men are.

Could the Japanese just happen to have unusually cancer-resistant prostate glands? Probably not, according to a report published in the *International Journal of Cancer;* in a study that compared the prostate glands from American, South American, Japanese, and Japanese-American men, Dr. R. Yatani, the lead researcher, found that Japanese men had almost as many latent, small, or benign prostate tumors as the men from the other countries had—but that these tumors just hadn't grown fast enough to become deadly. Perhaps some factor in the Japanese diet prevents the accelerated growth that is common to prostate tumors in American men. Could that anti-cancer factor be brewing in a cup of green tea?[20]

Investigators from the Cancer Research Center at the University of Chicago discovered that EGCG from green tea inhibited the growth of prostate tumors and also reduced the size of existing tumors. "It is possible that there is a relationship between the high consumption of green tea and the low incidence of prostate and breast cancers in some Asian countries," the researchers concluded.[21]

A precursor to prostate cancer is a condition called prostate intraepithelial neoplasia (PIN), and 30 percent of men with high grade PIN will develop prostate cancer within a year. Researchers in Italy worked with sixty men recently diagnosed with high grade PIN, and in a double blind study, gave half of them a placebo and the other half daily supplements of green tea catechins (600 milligrams per day).[22] As expected, 30 percent of the placebo users went on to develop prostate cancer. However, only 3 percent of those taking green tea extract developed a tumor.

Liver Cancer

Most tumors that form in the liver are malignant and are usually the result of cancers from other sites of the body that metastasize to the liver. Cancer can originate in the liver, but it is much less common than metastasized tumors. Liver cancer is more than twice as frequent in men than in women. Unfortunately, the majority of cases of liver cancer are fatal. Dr. James Klaunig from the Indiana University School of Medicine in Indianapolis suggests that green tea extract may show some promise in the prevention of liver cancer. He found that liver cells of treated mice have less free radical damage, improved gap junction communication, and healthier DNA replication, three conditions that contribute to a lesser risk of liver cancer, even in the face of carcinogens that target the liver.[23]

Pancreatic Cancer

Although many more people are stricken with cancers of the lung, colon, and breast, pancreatic cancer is a major killer. Most people who are diagnosed with cancer of the pancreas do not live more than six months. This poor survival rate is a result of the cancer's fast progression and a lack of effective treatments. Since treatment is not likely to inhibit pancreatic cancer, prevention is of primary importance. Although the evidence for green tea and pancreatic cancer is only preliminary, it is worth noting here since treatment options remain limited.[24] A study of 305 people in Poland (including pancreatic cancer cases and cancer-free controls) produced results suggesting that there is a "strongly significant trend of decreasing risk [of cancer of the pancreas] with increasing lifetime consumption of tea." Researchers who conducted a cohort study involving 13,979 residents of retirement homes in Los Angeles concluded that the "risk of pancreatic cancer decreased with increasing tea consumption." Yet another study, based on 213 pancreatic cancer patients and a cancer-free comparison group, revealed "significantly decreased risk" for those drinking green tea.[25]

Bladder Cancer

Approximately 67,000 new cases of bladder cancer are diagnosed annually, with four times as many men as women falling victim to the disease. Environmental factors play a role in cancer of the bladder, with cases much more common in cigarette smokers and industrial workers (including the dye, chemical, leather, and rubber industries). Polyphenols may mitigate some of the harmful effects of tobacco use. The International Agency for Research on Cancer determined that smokers with a high intake of polyphenols "are partially protected against the harmful effects of tobacco carcinogens within their bladder mucosal cells." Another study, involving 293 bladder cancer patients and 589 healthy controls, found that drinking green tea corresponded to a significantly lower risk of bladder cancer in women.[26] Even so, the overall evidence of green tea and bladder cancer remains equivocal. At this time, green tea cannot be clearly linked to a positive role in prevention or treatment of this cancer.[27]

Breast and Ovarian Cancers

These types of cancers are discussed in chapter 9.

Cancer Treatments

Cancer is no longer an automatic death sentence; in fact, most people diagnosed with cancer do not die from it, and the probability of a complete cure or extended survival is continually improving as scientists and physicians have a growing knowledge and understanding of cancer. For example, 63 percent of people survive colon cancer, 88 percent survive breast cancer, and 99 percent survive prostate cancer. Between the new tests that diagnose cancer at its earliest stages and the many successful therapies for cancer, things have never looked brighter for cancer patients.

There are three common qualities of all cancers, whether they strike the lung, prostate, skin, or any other organ or tissue of the body. These are:

- continued enlargement of the tumor through the ability of cancer cells to proliferate indefinitely
- invasion of the tumor into surrounding normal tissue
- tendency to metastasize to other parts of the body and establish new tumors

The goal of cancer treatments is the inhibition of these processes, that is, uncontrolled growth, tissue invasion, and metastasis.

Surgery was the first established treatment for cancer, and it remains the most widely used approach to dealing with cancer. Cancer surgery may have one or more of the following goals:

- to determine whether a cancer is malignant by biopsy examination
- to remove a cancerous growth from the body
- to learn whether malignant cells have spread to other parts of the body

Surgery is most effective in cases in which the cancer has not spread. This is most effectively associated with early detection.

Radiation therapy, in which a specific dose of high-energy X-rays or gamma rays is aimed at cancer cells to kill them selectively, is part of an overall cancer-treatment plan for the majority of cancer patients. It can be used in combination with surgery to shrink a tumor before surgery or to stop the growth of cancer cells that may remain after surgery. Healthy cells are better able to recover from radiation exposure than cancerous cells; consequently, radiation therapy can leave healthy parts of the body comparatively undamaged. An additional advantage of radiation over surgery is its ability to destroy tiny pockets of cancerous growth that the surgeon's knife might miss. Radiation also has less traumatic effects on older, frailer patients who might have a difficult time recovering from surgery and anesthesia. However, radiation therapy shares with surgery the shortcoming of sometimes failing to eradicate all the cancer cells of a tumor, and it cannot treat widespread metastasis or tumors that are not localized, such as leukemia, upon which the radiation cannot be focused. Also, radiation can cause many side effects, including nausea, hair loss, diarrhea, fatigue, and altered white blood cell levels, so it is difficult for the patient.

Chemotherapy, the systemic use of anti-cancer drugs that travel throughout the body via the blood vessels, is used in combination with surgery or radiation or both, depending on the severity of a case. Many chemotherapeutic drugs are used in combination, and new chemotherapeutic agents are added to the arsenal all the time. Unfortunately, just as bacteria can become resistant to antibiotics, some tumors become resistant to chemotherapeutic drugs. When this happens, the physician treating the patient must substitute another type of drug for the one that the cancer is now able to resist. When a tumor develops a resistance to multiple drugs, the problem is particularly serious, for the therapist's choices are fewer.

Many chemotherapeutic drugs fail because they also kill healthy cells in the body, causing serious side effects; this tendency limits the dosages that cancer doctors can give their patients. Commonly, chemotherapy drugs damage normal cells in the bone marrow, digestive tract, reproductive system, and hair follicles because these cells are dividing nearly as rapidly as tumor cells, although the damaged cells often recover after treatment is suspended. Other side effects caused by chemotherapy can include hair loss, mouth sores, nausea, vomiting, abnormal blood profiles, suppression of the immune response, and difficulty swallowing. Slow growing cancers, such as bowel cancers, are especially hard to treat in part because they grow slower than most tumors.

A chemotherapy drug called adriamycin (ADR) is one of the most effective broad-spectrum chemotherapy agents, but the dosage in which it can be used is limited because it also causes heart damage. One way to circumvent this type of toxicity problem is to combine a lower dosage of the chemotherapeutic drug with another agent that enhances the drug's effectiveness and minimizes its adverse effects. Dr. Yasuyuki Sadzuka and fellow cancer investigators from the University of Shizuoka, Japan, performed a novel study to determine whether green tea could contribute to more effective use of ADR. Dr. Sadzuka's research was based on theanine, an amino acid found primarily in green tea. At the start of his research, he pointed out that claims for the chemopreventive properties of green tea had already been backed by research, but this would be one of the first studies to reveal whether green tea is also a valuable adjunct in the treatment of cancer.[28]

Treating cancer cells growing in laboratory dishes with a combination of ADR and theanine resulted in higher concentrations of the chemotherapy drug within the tumor cells than did treatment with ADR alone. In animals, ADR alone shrinks tumors by 25 percent, but the ADR-and-theanine combination doubled this rate, achieving tumor shrinkage of 54 percent. Amazingly, the theanine appeared to enhance the effectiveness of the chemotherapy agent more than twofold, yet ADR levels in the heart (the main site of side effects) were reduced by 44 percent. These results indicate that theanine from green tea boosts the effectiveness of chemotherapy while minimizing its side effects. Dr. Sadzuka, summing up his research, commented that "it is confirmed that combination of theanine is able to enhance the anti-tumor activity without the increase of side effects of ADR."

The possibility of green tea as a supportive agent during cancer treatment first emerged in the minds of researchers as a result of the exposure of Japanese civilians to massive levels of radiation after the atomic bombings of Nagasaki and Hiroshima. Later, during the 1970s, Chinese investigators started to examine the potential of green tea extract as a protective agent against the effects of ionizing radiation. In 1994, several departments of the Second Affiliated Hospital of the Zhe Jiang Medical University began a clinical trial of green tea polyphenols.

Doctors in this hospital's Department of Oncology reported that tea polyphenols boosted the immune function of cancer patients, particularly in patients undergoing surgery or chemotherapy. These doctors recounted a typical breast cancer case, involving a woman named Wang. After an operation on her right breast, she required chemotherapy. During the course of chemotherapy, her white blood cell counts dropped. (White blood cells play many crucial roles in a healthy immune system.) Despite the administration of several drugs to correct her plummeting white blood cell count, it remained abnormally low. Her doctors then gave her daily green tea–polyphenol supplements. Within two weeks her white blood cell levels began to return to normal, and she was able to complete her full course of chemotherapy. Wang continued to take the polyphenol supplements after cancer treatment as a preventive measure. A single case is hardly convincing as proof, but it is nonetheless interesting.

A clinical investigation of the possible benefits of green tea polyphenols for radiation and chemotherapy patients was conducted at the Hu Nan province Hospital of Carcinology in China. This unpublished study involved sixty cancer patients; of these, twenty had cancer of the nasopharyngeal area, twenty had lung cancer, eight had breast cancer, and the remaining seven had cancers of the head or neck. All of these patients were undergoing their first round of radiation or chemotherapy and showed normal blood profiles before the initiation of cancer treatment.

These cancer patients were randomly placed in one of three groups:

- the polyphenol group, which received daily supplements of tea polyphenols from the first day of radiation or chemotherapy for one month
- the standard treatment group, which received the usual medication for improving blood quality
- the control group, which was not given any special medications throughout radiation or chemotherapy

The results were very promising. Throughout radiation or chemotherapy, the white blood cell counts remained stable for the group taking the tea polyphenols. In contrast, the cancer patients receiving the regular medication showed decreasing numbers of white blood cells during cancer treatment, and the control group had very significant drops in their numbers of white blood cells. The doctors concluded that the green tea extract "has a definite effect on the protection of the hemogram [blood profile] of patients undergoing radiation and chemotherapy, at least it is better than the common blood cell raising drug."[29]

Other hospitals in China were involved in another unpublished study to investigate the effectiveness of tea polyphenols in cancer patients who already had low white blood cell levels. The study observed forty-five patients who suffered from a variety of illnesses; their average age was fifty-one (with a range from nineteen to seventy-three years old).

The abnormal blood counts of the thirty-one patients who had cancer (including cancers of stomach, breast, lung, cervix, liver, and nasopharynx), were presumed to be a result of radiation therapy and chemotherapy. The abnormal white blood cell counts in the other patients were due to other conditions, including kidney and liver diseases. Most of the patients (forty-two out of forty-five) had already tried improving their blood status with one conventional therapy or another, to no avail.

After taking green tea extract supplements for thirty days, 60 percent of the patients had white blood cell counts increased by more than 50 percent, and another 31 percent had white blood cell counts increased by 30 to 50 percent. Some cases reported a complete reversal of abnormal blood counts in as short a time as seven days. Even after the supplements were suspended, blood counts remained normal for at least another two months. No side effects from treatment were reported. The doctors noted that while patients who had low white blood cell counts as a result of chemotherapy showed a good response to polyphenols, patients whose low counts were the result of radiation therapy showed a spectacular 100-percent response to polyphenols.[30] Further studies are under way to continue this line of investigation. Meanwhile, the encouraging preliminary results indicate that green tea, and the polyphenols derived from green tea, can be very supportive for cancer patients undergoing the difficult treatments of radiation and chemotherapy.

It seems clear that green tea is a powerful way to help prevent cancer, particularly for cancers afflicting the skin, gastrointestinal tract, lung, prostate, liver, pancreas, and bladder. In addition, green tea can play a supportive role during the treatment of cancer with radiation or chemotherapy. Of course, the promising story of green tea in cancer therapy is far from over; scientists continue to design and conduct research to clarify the benefits of green tea in cancer prevention and treatment. In the following chapter, we will turn our attention to green tea's ability to prevent another major killer: heart disease.

chapter six

Tea's Effect on Cardiovascular Disease

Cardiovascular disease takes the lives of almost one million Americans each year, more than any other disease. It's no surprise that people want to prevent and treat this deadly killer. Scientists, physicians, and patients have all made some progress. In one ten-year period, 1993 to 2003, death rates from all forms of cardiovascular disease declined by about 22 percent. Still, much more remains to be done for the one in three Americans who will eventually develop some form of cardiovascular disease. The old adage "An ounce of prevention is worth a pound of cure" certainly rings true in the case of heart disease. Keeping the heart and blood vessels in good shape is your best defense against developing heart disease. Along with a program of regular exercise and a healthful diet, green tea can play a valuable role in a heart disease prevention plan, since it lowers cholesterol levels, reduces blood pressure, and decreases the risk of heart attack and stroke.

The Causes of Heart Disease

Cardiovascular diseases comprise a large number of conditions affecting the heart and blood vessels, including atherosclerosis (hardening of the arteries), heart attack, and stroke. The condition that commonly comes to mind when discussing cardiovascular disease is *coronary artery disease,* which interrupts blood flow to the heart and can cause a heart attack.

Although the heart is a muscle full of blood, which it pumps throughout the body, it requires its own veins and arteries to supply it with nutrients and energy and to remove waste products. The coronary arteries and veins serve this function. If, for some reason, the coronary arteries do not deliver sufficient blood to the heart, a condition called *angina pectoralis* can develop. Stroke is a consequence of a similar interruption of blood supply to the brain. Either decrease in blood supply is usually traced to a blockage of key arteries by blood clots or cholesterol plaque.

In addition to clogging the arteries, another dangerous aspect of cardiovascular disease is atherosclerosis (hardening of the arteries). When the heart beats it delivers a large amount of blood into the arteries. These swell to receive the blood and, because they are normally elastic, they contract again. The contraction pushes against the heart valve that prevents blood from flowing back into the heart, and the blood is squeezed on its way around the body. When atherosclerosis is present, however, this normal distension and contraction becomes more difficult and blood pressure rises, placing excessive pressure on the heart. In some circumstances the blood vessels can even burst. Cholesterol is strongly implicated in this vascular problem.

The main symptoms of cardiovascular disease are:

- an abnormally uncomfortable awareness of breathing
- fatigue and weariness
- cough
- cyanosis (pale, ashen, or blue skin color)
- chest discomfort or pain
- palpitations, dizziness, or fainting
- swelling due to water retention
- pain or tiredness of calf muscles after exercise

Early research identified risk factors for cardiovascular disease by searching for common traits and lifestyles in people afflicted with the disease. These risk factors include:

- being male
- advancing age

- a family history of heart disease
- elevated blood cholesterol levels
- elevated homocysteine levels
- hypertension (high blood pressure)
- use of tobacco
- diabetes
- obesity
- stress
- use of oral contraceptives
- excessive alcohol intake
- malnutrition
- lack of physical activity

More than 90 percent of cardiovascular patients have been found to have prior exposure to at least one of these cardiovascular disease risk factors. So the good news is that finding out which risk factors you have, and modifying any that you can, makes a huge potential difference to your future health.

Cholesterol stands center stage as one of the most important risk factors in the development of cardiovascular diseases. Knowing cholesterol's reputation, many people are surprised to find out that cholesterol is produced by our bodies naturally and performs many functions essential for health. For example, cholesterol is a building block for steroid hormones, such as sexual hormones and cortisone, it is converted into vitamin D when the skin is exposed to sunlight, and it is involved in the biosynthesis of bile salts, which are important for the intestinal absorption of fats. Cholesterol is also important during the metabolism of carbohydrates and acts as a vehicle to transport fat-soluble vitamins (such as vitamins A and E and beta-carotene) in the bloodstream. It also supplies material for building cell membranes, especially in nervous tissue. Thus it is necessary in the right proportions for the maintenance of health.

Cholesterol first acquired its bad rap as an instigator of heart disease all the way back in 1913. That's when a Russian scientist named Nikolai Anitschkow fed a group of rabbits a very high-cholesterol diet as an experiment. When Anitschkow examined the rabbits' blood vessels, he found them to be hardened and clogged with plaque, a condition known as atherosclerosis. Hardened arteries are less elastic than youthful, healthy arteries and contribute to poor circulation and high blood pressure. Since the addition of cholesterol to their diet was the only significant experimental change in the lives of these animals, Anitschkow concluded that cholesterol was the cause of their cardiovascular disease.

Researchers subsequently hypothesized that more cholesterol in the diet translated into more cholesterol in the blood. This extra cholesterol settles onto the blood vessel walls to form deposits of fatty plaque that may build up until they eventually block the normal flow of blood. If a clot forms where a deposit of plaque has accumulated, blood flow can be completely blocked, causing a heart attack or stroke. The heart is the one muscle in the body that can never rest, so an uninterrupted supply of nutrients and removal of waste products is essential to it. The very large energy requirements of the brain also require an uninterrupted blood flow for normal functioning.

The relationship between cholesterol and heart disease is not clearcut; there are some uncertainties. For example, most of the cholesterol in the bloodstream is manufactured by the liver, not extracted from cholesterol-rich foods. In fact, only about one-third of blood cholesterol can be traced to dietary sources, and a number of researchers have pointed out that for this reason avoiding cholesterol-rich foods has only a limited effect on lowering total cholesterol levels. However, other dietary factors, particularly the amount of saturated fat in the diet, do influence cholesterol levels greatly.

In an effort to reconcile the uncertainties in the cholesterol theory of cardiovascular disease, many scientists have focused their attention on the roles of different types of lipoproteins that transport cholesterol and other fats through the bloodstream to various parts of the body. Low density lipoproteins transport the greatest percentage of the body's cholesterol, and they transfer some of it to artery walls, where it may accumulate as plaque. In contrast, high density lipoproteins shuttle excess cholesterol back to the liver, where it is broken down and excreted from the body in the bile. Cholesterol carried by low density lipoproteins is called, for short, LDL-cholesterol, and cholesterol carried by high density lipoproteins is called HDL-cholesterol. A relatively high level of LDL-cholesterol in the blood indicates a risk of accumulating arterial plaque, while a relatively high level of HDL-cholesterol may actually help prevent plaque buildup. Thus, the concept of LDL-cholesterol as the "bad

Cholesterol and Cardiovascular Disease

According to the National Cholesterol Education Program, the risk of cardiovascular disease varies with blood cholesterol levels. For instance, if your total cholesterol level is 200 and your HDL-cholesterol is 50, you have a ratio of 4.0 to 1, indicating a low to moderate risk of developing cardiovascular disease.[1]

	Low Risk	Moderate Risk	High Risk
Total cholesterol	Less than 200	200 to 239	More than 240
LDL-Cholesterol	Less than 130	130 to 159	More than 160
HDL-Cholesterol	More than 50	40 to 50	Less than 35
Ratio of Total to HDL	Below 3.5 to 1	4.5 to 1	6.5 to 1

* All measurements are in milligrams per deciliter of blood. These categories apply to adults age 20 and above.

cholesterol" and HDL-cholesterol as the "good cholesterol" was born. In this view, the total level of blood cholesterol is less important than how well it is mobilized or expelled.

Scientists have theorized that the ratio between different cholesterols is a more important indication of the risk of cardiovascular disease than is the total cholesterol level alone. To prevent cardiovascular diseases, public health officials have urged people to decrease LDL-cholesterol as a percentage of total blood cholesterol and increase the percentage of the total represented by HDL-cholesterol. (See the table above for risk levels associated with various cholesterol levels.) You should have your blood cholesterol levels checked at least once every five years.

Unfortunately, just keeping tabs on your cholesterol levels and ratios is not necessarily a sure-fire way to avoid cardiovascular disease. Heart attacks often strike men and women with apparently "normal" cholesterol levels and ratios. Doctors with patients who had enviably low cholesterol levels, yet still suffered heart attacks or other cardiovascular diseases concluded, understandably, that cholesterol levels were not the full explanation. Pieces of the cardiovascular disease puzzle were obviously missing.

In the continued search for the missing factors, some researchers focused on the effects of free radical damage to cholesterol. Numerous studies indicate that LDL-cholesterol is one of the prime targets of free radicals, and once LDL-cholesterol is oxidized it becomes a very nasty substance. Scientists had already implicated nonoxidized LDL-cholesterol in the initiation of atherosclerosis; now they realized that oxidized LDL-cholesterol was even more likely to damage blood vessels and promote cardiovascular disease. Antioxidants show a great deal of promise in preventing the oxidation of LDL-cholesterol and thus reducing this cardiovascular disease risk factor.[2]

The French Paradox and the Green Tea Connection

The story of green tea and a healthy heart actually begins, not in Asia, but in France, with the French Paradox, the medical oddity that we discussed in Chapter 3. The French Paradox results from the fact that the French outlive Americans and suffer significantly fewer heart attacks, despite the fact that smoking is a national pastime in France and the typical French diet is swimming in saturated fat. It just didn't seem to make sense that the French would have healthy hearts despite the double whammy of smoking and saturated fat. The answer seems to lie in the red wine swirling in French wine glasses, wine that is an excellent source of polyphenols (the same class of nutrients to which green tea's active ingredients belong). As antioxidants, red wine's polyphenols are believed to mitigate the effects of a fatty diet and smoking.[3]

A similar paradox is seen in Japan. Despite a high percentage of smokers (estimated to be as much as 75 percent of adult men), Japan has an astonishingly low rate of heart disease. It seems possible that the polyphenols in green tea cause the same paradox that those in red wine lead to. In fact, laboratory studies of animals show that even in the face of a high-fat diet, green tea prevents atherosclerosis in animals. A similar effect has been documented in people. Even when subjects ate three egg yolks every day, the concurrent consumption of green tea kept blood cholesterol levels in the normal range, despite the massive amounts of cholesterol present in the egg yolks.[4]

One of the largest epidemiological studies to investigate the relationship of diet to heart disease is the Seven Countries Study. A total of 12,763 middle-aged men from seven countries were enrolled in this study between 1958 and 1964 and followed for the next twenty-five years to track mortality from any cause, but heart disease in particular. Dietary assessments in these men showed that intake of flavonoids varied greatly from country to country. (Flavonoids are naturally occurring compounds, found in many plants and foods, that have antioxidant, disease-preventing effects.) In Finland, only 2.6 milligrams of flavonoids daily were consumed, while in Japan the average was 68.2 milligrams daily (80 percent of them derived from green tea). According to Dr. Michael Hertog from the National Institute of Public and Environmental Protection, Bilthoven, the Netherlands, the greater the intake of flavonoids, the lesser the risk of heart disease in these men. The mortality rates from heart disease varied greatly between the seven countries in this study, and the differences in flavonoid intake accounted for one-quarter of these differences.[5]

As an extension of the Seven Countries Study, Dr. Hertog conducted a more in-depth analysis of the Netherlands arm of the study. The flavonoid intake of 805 elderly men was compared with their risk for cardiovascular diseases over a five-year period. The primary sources of flavonoids in this population were tea (61 percent), onions (13 percent), and apples (10 percent). During the observation period, forty-three men died of coronary heart disease. The volume of flavonoids in their diets was inversely related to the likelihood of death from heart disease; that is, as flavonoid intake went up, the risk of fatal heart attack went down. Nonfatal heart attacks were also inversely related to consumption of flavonoids. The risk of heart disease for the men with the highest intake of flavonoids was half that of the men with the lowest intake.[6]

A Few Cups a Day to Protect the Heart

According to a recent study of 40,530 Japanese adults, those who drank the most green tea (compared to those drinking much less) were less likely to die from cardiovascular disease.[7] These individuals were followed for seven years. The women drinking five-plus cups daily had a 31 percent lower risk of dying from cardiovascular disease (compared to women drinking one or less cups daily) and the men in the green tea–loving group had a reduced risk of 22 percent. In addition, green tea reduced the risk of clot-related strokes. For the women in the five-plus cup group it was 62 percent lower risk of dying from these strokes and it was a 42 percent lower risk for the men.

An interesting aside: Because tea drinking is popular in Japan across economic levels and differing lifestyles, this study seems to indicate that green tea provides health benefits above and beyond just being correlated with people who tend to make other good health choices. In other words, some people in the past wondered if green tea was healthy in and of itself, or it was just a coincidence that health-conscious people (that is, those who exercise, eat their veggies, etc.) happen to also drink tea. This study indicates that green tea is healthy regardless of other healthy choices you may or may not be making.

Researchers from the University of North Carolina School of Public Health conducted a meta-analysis to get a better understanding about the role of tea in heart health.[8] A meta-analysis is a type of study that pools together data from many other studies—in this case seventeen prior studies. Individually, each study may be too small to show significant results, but taken as a whole, the findings would be weightier.

Here's the short version of what this meta-analysis discovered: Drinking just three cups of tea each day can decrease the risk of heart attack by 11 percent. The studies included in the meta-analysis were looking into the risk of either heart attack, stroke, or coronary heart disease (narrowing of the blood vessels feeding the heart). When the researchers sliced-and-diced the numbers in different ways, they determined that drinking an additional three cups of tea daily can lower the occurrence of both heart attack and coronary heart disease by a whopping two-thirds.

Additional evidence for the positive role of tea for the heart comes from a seven-year study of U.S. women reporting that the risk of important vascular events (heart attack, stroke, or death from cardiovascular disease) was significantly lower in women who drank at least four cups tea per day.[9]

The Effect of Green Tea on Cholesterol Levels

Research based on flavonoids strongly suggests a relationship between green tea and reduction of heart disease, but you needn't make a leap of faith from the effects of flavonoids in general to the effects of green tea's polyphenols, because there's ample direct evidence in the literature dealing specifically with green tea. For example, a Japanese epidemiologist, Dr. K. Imai, interviewed 1,371 men aged forty and older to gather information about their diet, lifestyle, and average daily consumption of green tea. He also analyzed their blood with several biochemical assays. Drinking green tea turned out to be strongly indicative of lower levels of cholesterol, even after taking into account age, smoking, alcohol use, and body weight. Men who drank ten or more cups of green tea daily had significantly lower cholesterol levels. The cholesterol profile was favorably affected in the green tea drinkers, and LDL-cholesterol (the bad cholesterol) decreased while HDL-cholesterol (the good cholesterol) increased in those who drank the most green tea.

Free-radical damage to blood vessels, which is a contributing factor to the initiation of atherosclerosis, can be measured by the levels of lipid peroxides in the blood. Because of the numerous free radicals in tobacco smoke, smokers have much higher lipid peroxide levels than nonsmokers; which partially accounts for the increased risk of heart disease in smokers. Accordingly, Dr. Imai found that lipid peroxides were greatly increased in the subset of his study population comprising men who smoked. However, heavy smokers who were also among the most dedicated green tea drinkers (more than ten cups daily) had lipid peroxide profiles similar to nonsmokers. The green tea was able to counteract the damaging effects of tobacco use, and the decreased levels of this marker of tobacco use attested to the beneficial effect of the tea.[10]

Researchers from the U.S. Department of Agriculture looked into the influence of tea on a small group of adults with mildly elevated cholesterol following a "Step I" type diet. This diet, developed by the American Heart Association and the National Cholesterol Education Program, is moderately low in fat and cholesterol. As an additional effort to aid cholesterol levels, participants drank five cups of tea daily for three weeks. After this short amount of time, the combination of diet changes and tea drinking lowered LDL cholesterol by 11 percent and total cholesterol by 6.5 percent.[11]

Another group of Japanese researchers reported similar good news about green tea. At the International Symposium on Physiological and Pharmacological Effects of *Camellia sinensis* (Tea): Implications for Cardiovascular Disease, Cancer, and Public Health, Dr. Suminori Kono and fellow researchers announced that health examinations of 1,306 retiring government officials indicated that consuming green tea lowered cholesterol levels. The men who regularly drank nine cups of green tea or more daily had total cholesterol levels that were 8 milligrams per deciliter lower than the men who drank two cups or less daily.[12] This effect is not dramatic, but it is a change in the right direction.

At the same symposium, scientists from the University of Oslo, Norway, presented data gathered halfway around the world from the site of the Japanese study, yet producing nearly identical results. According to the health facts of approximately 20,000 middle-aged Norwegian men and women, cholesterol levels decrease as (black) tea consumption increases. Men drinking five or more cups of tea daily had total cholesterol levels 9.3 milligrams per deciliter lower than those drinking one cup or less daily, and women had levels 5.8 milligrams per deciliter lower. Furthermore, people who did not drink tea were more likely to die from a heart attack than tea drinkers were. The results of this study are all the more impressive when we consider that Norwegians drink black tea, which contains much lower levels of polyphenols than green tea does.[13]

A study of 5,369 employees of twenty-one Israeli factories also focused on a population that primarily drank black tea. Besides the use of black tea instead of the more health-protecting green tea in Israel, there were very few tea drinkers of any sort in this study population. Nonetheless, as the daily number of cups of tea grew, total cholesterol levels shrank. There was also a trend toward lower LDL-cholesterol levels and higher HDL-cholesterol levels in these men and women.[14]

With the evidence indicating a preventive effect for green tea in the risk of cardiovascular disease mounting, it would be interesting to find out *how* green tea helps defeat one of the world's most dangerous killers. The antioxidant capability of green tea definitely tops the list. As discussed earlier, the oxidation of LDL-cholesterol creates an especially dangerous substance, in terms of initiating blood vessel damage and atherosclerosis. As antioxidants, green tea's polyphenols help prevent this damage. When scientists cultured LDL-cholesterol cells in the laboratory, they confirmed that EGCG almost completely inhibited free radical damage to LDL-cholesterol.[15] L-theanine, an amino acid found almost exclusively in green tea, is another component of green tea that is responsible for lessening the dangerous oxidation of LDL cholesterol.[16]

There is an even more basic mechanism used by green tea to reduce the risk of heart disease: blocking the absorption of cholesterol. If cholesterol from the diet is not able to enter the body, then it will not increase blood cholesterol levels. To clarify this protective effect of green tea, researchers from the Laboratory of Nutrition Chemistry at the Kyushu University School of Agriculture in Japan set up a series of animal experiments. Groups of rats were fed diets rich in cholesterol and saturated fat, with and without the addition of various green tea polyphenols. The absorption of cholesterol was markedly inhibited by the polyphenols, with the most effective cholesterol inhibitor being EGCG. Consequently, blood cholesterol levels were correspondingly lower, as well. Rats fed a diet based on cholesterol and coconut oil absorbed 48.5 percent of the cholesterol, but simply adding EGCG to this diet reduced cholesterol absorption to 16.7 percent.

These investigators then set out to determine how EGCG blocked the absorption of cholesterol. They discovered that EGCG joined with bile salt and emulsified cholesterol to form an insoluble precipitate that cannot be absorbed by the intestine and is therefore excreted in the feces. It was suggested that "since EGCG is a major component of catechins in Japanese green tea, the amount of catechins in green tea taken after a meal seems possible to precipitate dietary cholesterol" and prevent its absorption from that meal.[17]

Heart Attack

Drinking about three cups of tea each day seems to be the key number for significant heart health benefits. This amount has been shown in research to reduce the risk of having a heart attack and lower LDL ("bad") cholesterol levels. People who drank 16 ounces (that's two cups) of black tea per day were found to have a 50 percent lower prevalence of heart disease than non–tea drinkers, according to researchers in Saudi Arabia.[18] This study of 3,430 men and women adjusted for other risk factors, such as age and smoking.

And in another interesting study, drinking three or more cups of black tea daily slashes the risk of having a heart attack by a whopping 43 percent, compared to non–tea drinkers.[19] An earlier study by this same set of Dutch researchers had found that people who drank one to two cups of tea daily lowered their risk of severe hardening of the aortic artery by 46 percent. And those tea lovers who drank more than four cups every day had a 69 percent lower risk of this condition, which is a strong indicator of cardiovascular disease.[20]

When researchers at Harvard examined the lives of 340 men and women who had a heart attack and compared them with heart-healthy controls, they found some very interesting patterns. The people who drank even just a cup of black tea a day (and some drank more than a cup daily) had a 44 percent lower risk of heart attack compared to non–tea drinkers.[21] And in another Harvard study, this time involving 1,900 people, researchers discovered that those who drank tea in the year before they had a heart attack were more than 40 percent more likely to survive the heart attack and still be alive during the following three years that they were tracked by this study.[22]

And finally, when Australian researchers combined the data from numerous studies, they were able to compare the dietary habits of 2,087 people who died from a fatal heart attack to the dietary habits of people without heart disease. Individuals who were in the top third of flavonol intake (with tea accounting for the bulk of these nutrients) had a 20 percent lesser chance of dying from a heart attack than those in the bottom third of flavonol intake.[23]

The Prevention of Unhealthy Blood Clots

Aside from abnormally high cholesterol levels, other factors contribute to the development of atherosclerosis and, potentially, to a heart attack. Abnormal clotting of the blood is one such factor. The blood's ability to form clots is very important; without clots, bleeding from a cut or torn blood vessel could continue unchecked and ultimately lead to death. To stop excessive blood loss in such a situation, the blood vessel contracts in a spasm (to limit the amount of blood that can escape), and blood platelets (tiny disc-shaped cells) bunch together to form a plug or, if the injury is severe, a blood clot. Thromboxane, a modified type of fatty acid circulating in the bloodstream, is released during blood vessel injuries and is responsible for initiating a decrease in blood flow and the release of additional blood clotting factors.

Of course, the body has to have a way to control the clotting process; if it did not, the entire circulatory system could become clotted. This is why the blood also contains anti-clotting factors. Sometimes, however, the sequence of events leading to blood clotting is initiated when it isn't needed; in these cases, a blood clot can form along the wall of a blood vessel and increase the risk of heart attack or stroke. Again, it is important to minimize this potential damage with anti-clotting mechanisms. Although the blood makes anti-clotting factors itself, some dietary substances can also reduce the possibility of undesired blood clotting. One of these dietary substances is green tea. Green tea inhibits the formation of thromboxane, and a low level of thromboxane in turn inhibits blood clots.[24] Laboratory research indicates that rats given green tea extract have significantly lower thromboxane levels; this beneficial effect is not seen with processed black tea extract.[25] Other studies in animals confirm that green tea lessens the clotting tendency and prevents platelet aggregation.[26] Some research even suggests that EGCG is as effective as aspirin, the well known and commonly used anticoagulant, or "blood thinner."[27] Those who need a stronger anti-clotting agent should consult a physician.

Chinese doctors report favorable results using dietary supplements of green tea polyphenols to diminish rates of occurrence of heart disease. Forty patients with a variety of cardiovascular diseases (including coronary heart disease and hypertension) were found to have in common the problem of excessive fibrinogen levels. (Fibrinogen is a blood protein involved in the cascade of events that leads to blood clotting.) Excessive fibrinogen levels lead to abnormally high tendencies to form blood clots. After suspending the use of anti-clotting medications and substituting daily supplements of polyphenols, all of the patients showed reductions in their abnormally high tendency to form blood clots. Presumably, this improvement would reduce their risk of heart attack or stroke.

Doctors treating heart disease patients at the First Hospital of Zhe

Jiang Medical University in China were also pleased with the beneficial effects of green tea polyphenols. High levels of fibrinogen were found in 100 patients with coronary heart disease, history of heart attack, angina pectoris, history of stroke, or hypertension. After a month's course of treatment with polyphenol supplements, 95 percent of the patients experienced significant reductions in their abnormal tendency toward forming blood clots.

Another set of patients, seen at the First People's Hospital of Xiao Shan City in China, was treated with green tea polyphenols after being diagnosed with angina pectoris, a condition characterized by attacks of chest pain, usually brought on by physical exertion. Angina is often a symptom of atherosclerosis and can be a warning sign of future heart attacks. Fourteen of the twenty-eight patients also had high fibrinogen levels. After a month's course of supplementation with green tea extract, the doctors reported that angina attacks were controlled in 71 percent of the patients. In addition, fibrinogen levels were reduced in all but one patient and electrocardiogram results normalized in fifteen of the patients. Angina patients are usually prescribed powerful medication for this condition, and they should continue taking that medication. Although the evidence available today supports the likelihood that green tea polyphenols can help prevent or modulate the severity of developing angina, extracts of green tea polyphenols are not a substitute for medication when angina has developed.

Flexible Blood Vessels

Yet another way that tea helps the cardiovascular system is by improving blood vessel function, specifically by allowing blood vessels to dilate, or open up, more to allow the blood to flow more easily when the body needs more blood. When a group of patients with coronary artery disease drank black tea, their blood vessels began to function more like healthy people.[28] Other research supports this finding, that regular drinking of tea improves blood vessel dilation. For example, when adults with mildly elevated cholesterol levels drank either five cups of black tea or hot water (as a control) every day for a month, those drinking tea were found to have improvements in the flexibility of their blood vessels.[29]

The Silent Epidemic of Hypertension

One out of every three adults in the United States has hypertension (high blood pressure), while another 59 million people has pre-hypertension (the early stages of this disease). Although effective therapy has been available for more than half a century, most people with hypertension do not have their blood pressure under control. Of the people who have hypertension, 36 percent do not know that they have the disorder, and only 29 percent have their high blood pressure adequately controlled.

In other words, a large majority of the people who have hypertension either are not aware of their condition or are not handling it successfully. However, hypertension is easily and painlessly diagnosed through a blood pressure test, and most hypertensives can lower and even normalize their blood pressure through dietary changes, exercise, and weight reduction. Powerful medications are available when these measures fail.

Hypertension is dangerous because the damage it does to blood vessel linings can lead to a series of severe pathologies, including atherosclerosis. The elevated arterial pressure also weakens the blood vessel walls, encouraging the development of aneurysms that diminish cardiovascular function and that, when ruptured, can cause stroke, internal bleeding, and a host of other life-threatening conditions. Congestive heart failure and damage to the kidneys are also common in uncontrolled hypertension.

One of the things that makes hypertension so serious is its lack of obviously unpleasant symptoms; it is a silent killer. Anxiety, heart poundings, or increased pulse rate are not necessarily indicators of high blood pressure. The only reliable way to detect abnormal pressure is to have a blood pressure check. The reading from a blood pressure test gives two numbers. The first number is called the systolic blood pressure, which is the greatest amount of pressure exerted against the walls of the arteries at any one time when the heart muscle is in the pumping phase. The second number, called the diastolic blood pressure, reflects the lower amount of pressure during the phase when the heart valve is closed and the elastic arteries squeeze the blood onward through the body. A normal blood pressure reading is 120/80 or less; in other words, the systolic pressure is 120 millimeters of mercury or less, and the diastolic pressure is 80 millimeters of mercury or less. Borderline high blood pressure falls in the range of 140/90 to 160/95. Hypertension is regarded as blood pressure greater than 160/95 in repeated measurements. Temporary or transient elevation in blood pressure can reflect anxiety, transient dietary factors, changes in exercise habits, and the like and may not reflect disease at all. Routinely high levels, however, are not normal and are signals to seek professional help.

No accurate set of predictors exists to indicate who will develop hypertension and who will not, other than our knowledge that certain populations, such as African Americans, have a higher incidence of hypertension. Interestingly, among people who are middle-aged or younger, more men than women have hypertension, but in the older population more women than men have the condition. Essential hypertension—hypertension for which the cause is unknown—accounts for more than 90 percent of the cases. We do know that blood pressure is affected by several factors, including body weight, certain dietary components, genetic predisposition, cigarette smoking, stress, exercise, and percentage of body fat. Endocrine disorders, including adult-onset diabetes associated with obesity, also contribute to hypertension.[30]

The Norwegian study of 20,000 middle-aged adults that we discussed earlier in terms of cholesterol levels also included data regarding blood pressure. Systolic blood pressure decreased steadily in both men and women as their average tea intake increased. Research conducted on animals revealed a similar inverse relationship between tea intake and blood pressure. When mice were subjected to stressful conditions, such as overcrowding, their blood pressure rose, but adding decaffeinated green tea to their water kept rising blood pressures in check, despite the mounting stress levels. Dr. Satoshi Umemura from the Yokohama City University School of Medicine in Japan, reported that green tea lowered blood pressure in rats with hypertension, but he found even better blood pressure-lowering effects with a green tea processed to make it especially rich in GABA, an inhibitory neurotransmitter involved with blood pressure regulation. (The processing involved oxidizing fresh tea leaves under nitrogen.) Dr. Umemura suggested that "because people in many countries have a habit of drinking tea, the administration of GABA-rich tea might become one of the supportive methods to decrease blood pressure in essential hypertension."[31] Normally prepared tea would have this property greatly diminished.

The unique amino acid found in green tea, called L-theanine, has been extracted from green tea and studied by itself and found to reduce blood pressure. This research remains in the animal model stage, but future studies in human populations should clarify whether L-theanine will have the same effect in people.

Relaxing the blood vessel walls can be helpful in hypertension. When Dr. David Fitzpatrick investigated the ability of dozens of plant extracts to relax blood vessels, he found that green tea came out near the top of the list. Out of the fifty-four vegetables, fruits, nuts, herbs, spices, and teas that he tested, green tea was ranked number five, producing a 91 percent relaxation of the endothelium (lining of blood vessels). Black tea, presumably because it has lower polyphenol levels, only relaxed the blood vessels by 66 percent.[32]

The "Brain Attacks" Called Strokes

Stroke is the third leading cause of death in the United States and a leading cause of serious, long-term disability. Strokes belong to a class of disorders called "cerebrovascular disease," meaning that the blood vessels feeding the brain are involved. Each year approximately 700,000 Americans suffer a stroke. Since a heart attack results from interrupted blood flow to the heart, we might say that a stroke is a "brain attack" in which the brain's blood flow is interrupted. Symptoms of a stroke can include sudden numbness, weakness, or paralysis; speaking difficulties; blurred vision; dizziness; and sudden, severe headaches. Atherosclerosis is the most common underlying cause of a stroke, since it can result in narrowing of the arteries and possible association with a blood clot that blocks blood flow to the brain. High cholesterol levels are a risk factor for strokes. It is estimated by cardiovascular disease experts that 70 percent of strokes occur in people with high blood pressure.

The meta-analysis from the University of North Carolina School of Public Health researchers mentioned earlier in this chapter also looked at the risk of stroke in tea drinkers and non–tea drinkers. For stroke, drinking three cups daily resulted in a 12 percent lower incidence. And the longer a person is a regular daily tea drinker, the stronger tea's protective effects. Specifically, for each year that one drinks tea, there is an additional 5 percent protection from having a stroke. Could protecting yourself from stroke be any easier or tastier?

In another extension of the Seven Countries Study mentioned earlier, researchers from the National Institute of Public Health and Environmental Protection in the Netherlands observed 552 Dutch men, aged fifty to sixty-nine, for fifteen years; among other things, the researchers monitored the incidence of stroke in the group. The men with the highest intake of flavonoids had 73 percent fewer strokes than the men with a low intake of flavonoids. Black tea provided 70 percent of the flavonoids in the diets of these men, and apples provided another 10 percent. When researchers analyzed the data for tea drinkers separately, they found that risk of experiencing a stroke was 69 percent lower for men who drank more than 4.7 cups of tea each day than for men who drank 2.6 cups or less daily. The lead researcher, Dr. Sirving Keli, suggested that the flavonoids protected against stroke by acting as antioxidants and preventing blood clots.[33]

Pursuing a similar line of inquiry, Japanese investigators gathered information about medical history and daily consumption of green tea from 5,910 women older than forty who neither smoked nor drank. They discovered that stroke was less common among the women who drank more green tea. Further data gathered from the women over the next four years showed that new cases of stroke or cerebral hemorrhage were twice as likely among the women who drank five cups of green tea or less daily than among the green tea lovers.[34]

A clinical trial conducted at the Beijing Ji Shui Tan Hospital in China was one of the first to examine the possible benefits of green tea polyphenols given to people *after* they had had a stroke. Forty patients were enrolled in the study—twenty-nine men and eleven women. Their average age was sixty-six. When each patient was admitted to the hospital, personnel graded the patient's health status according to the standards adopted by the Second National Conference on Cerebrovascular Disease. According to those standards, the effects of stroke were slight in twenty-eight of the patients, medium in nine patients, and severe in three. The same grading scale was used to reevaluate the patients' health after four weeks of daily doses of polyphenols extracted from green tea. Following this therapeutic regimen, surprising improvements were observed in the patients. Nine of the patients (23 percent) were basically cured, another 47 percent of the patients showed significant improvements, and 18 percent showed at least some progresses.[35]

Cardiovascular disease has been the number one killer in the United States every single year since 1900 (with the exception of 1918, during the flu pandemic). In this country, there is a death from cardiovascular disease every thirty-five seconds. In fact, cardiovascular disease claims more lives each year than the next four causes of death combined (cancer, chronic lower respiratory disease, accidents, and diabetes). If cardiovascular disease could be eliminated, life expectancy would jump by nearly seven years.

Green tea's polyphenols can help turn the tide against this loss of life. The following chapters will show the many ways in which green tea polyphenols also improve the quality of life, including detoxifying the body, boosting immune function, and keeping the teeth healthy.

chapter seven

Longevi-tea

Have you ever tried to read your fortune in tea leaves? Well, if you brewed green tea, those leaves might spell out a long life. Green tea has been promoted as a way to extend life since at least as long ago as 1211, when Eisai Myo-an, the founder of Zen Buddhism, wrote a book claiming that green tea maintains good health and prolongs life. Scientific proof has been a long time coming, but researchers are finally gathering support for Eisai's claim that green tea can lengthen the life span.

Getting older isn't what it used to be; the "baby boomer" generation is redefining the meaning of aging. No longer are men and women in their forties and fifties considered "over the hill"—especially not when a growing percentage of the population is living more than a century. More than 76 million Americans will be older than sixty-five by the year 2040, according to the U.S. Census Bureau; and that same decade will see a whopping 13 million living past the eighty-five-year mark. Number crunchers at Duke University see the future even more brightly: They predict 138 million senior citizens in 2040. And both predictions agree that centenarians are the fastest growing age group.

Most of us want to not only extend our life span but also to extend our "health span." Health span means living a healthy, active life for as long as possible. And green tea can help people do just that: live longer while living healthier.

Drinking Your Way to a Long Life

One reason for believing in green tea's life-enhancing qualities is the typical life span enjoyed by green tea–loving populations, including many of the Asian countries. Statistics show that Asians have a lower risk of contracting or dying from many of the diseases that plague our own country. Even after adjusting the statistics to account for factors that could affect health—such as access to medical care, smoking, genetic differences, and pollution—Asian countries still rank high in worldwide comparisons of longevity and health.

The Asian secret to a longer, healthier life appears to lie in dietary choices. Asian diets are well-known for what they *don't* contain: They are low in fat, meat, refined grains, and sugar. But what is served on the dinner tables in Japan and China, such as plenty of vegetables, complex carbohydrates, and soy foods, may be just as important as what's missing from them. More specifically, what's brewing in Asian teapots accounts for at least part of the secret to Asian longevity.

Green tea fanatics just plain live longer than people who avoid tea. One study that uncovered this fact examined the relationship of green tea to longevity by following the lives of 3,380 Japanese women for nine years. These women were all at least fifty years old and were all registered teachers of the Japanese tea ceremony in Tokyo. Green tea is an essential component of the Japanese tea ceremony, so the researchers assumed that these women were greater-than-average green tea drinkers. All deaths that occurred from 1980 to 1988 in this group were recorded. After comparing these numbers with the mortality rates of other Japanese women, within Tokyo and throughout Japan during the same time period, the researchers discovered that a smaller percentage of the green tea drinkers died, "indicating the possibility that green tea is a protective factor for several fatal diseases."[1]

The few laboratory studies that have considered the longevity of animals support a life-extending role for tea. Chinese researchers found that fruit flies, which generally live only fifteen days, stay alive a stunning forty days when jasmine tea is added to their drinking water. (Imagine the equivalent: the average human life span of seventy years would be extended to 186 years!) Japanese researchers at the Nagasaki University

Green Tea's Role in a Long, Healthy Life

This chart lists the "symptoms" or observable effects of aging, their physical causes, and the "counteractions" of green tea for each.

Barrier to Longevity	Green Tea Benefits
Heart Disease	Lowers cholesterol and blood pressure and prevents platelet aggregation.
Cancer	Inhibits the initiation, promotion, and progression of cancer.
Diabetes	Promotes normal blood sugar and insulin regulation.
Poor Nutrition	Indirectly linked to a better diet, since green tea drinkers tend to make healthier food choices.
Unhealthy Lifestyle	Indirectly associated with healthier lifestyles, since green tea drinkers are less likely to smoke and more likely to be physically active.
Weak Immune System	Bolsters immunity and has anti-microbial properties.
Environmental Toxins	Aids in the proper function of the liver, which helps detoxify the body.
Poor Mental Function	Promotes healthy cognitive functions; may help prevent senility.

School of Medicine had similar results in an experiment with rats. When rats were given EGCG in their water, their life span was considerably prolonged. The researchers who conducted this study identified the free radical–fighting abilities of green tea as its longevity-enhancing aspect.[2]

Most health experts agree that the "free radical theory of aging" holds the most promise for understanding—and slowing—the aging process. Free radical "hits" on cells and their essential components accumulate over time, resulting in deleterious alterations in cellular structure and decreasing the ability of enzymes to function, thus producing the signs and symptoms of aging: premature death, heart disease, cancer, dimming cognition, cataracts, and wrinkles. If free radicals are the problem, then antioxidants are, without a doubt, the solution. According to Dr. Denham Harman, a free radical expert from the University of Nebraska, "addition of one of a number of different antioxidants in the diet can increase the average life span." Undoubtedly, green tea's polyphenols are potent antioxidants that can help hold back the hands of time.[3]

Is the effort to increase longevity just a numbers game, with mankind trying to break the triple-digit mark? Does anyone really want to live past 100 if his or her last several decades are spent in a nursing home? Our true goal is probably better explained as the effort to increase the likelihood of "dying young as late as possible" by extending our "health span," not just our life span. There are many ways that green tea's polyphenols improve the quality of a person's health and extend the health span. For instance, as we reported in the preceding chapters, green tea helps prevent heart disease and cancer, which together are the top two killers of Americans and account for 60 percent of all deaths.

Green tea's potential as a protective agent against premature death from heart disease and cancer is impressive. Researchers have found that green tea's polyphenols bolster the heart's resistance to cardiovascular diseases by lowering levels of total cholesterol and LDL-cholesterol, reducing platelet aggregation, and helping keep blood pressure in check. As an agent in the prevention of cancer, green tea inhibits both the initiation and promotion stages of cancer and even boosts the effectiveness of some cancer treatments.

Free Radical Theory of Aging

For many years scientists struggled to unlock the mystery of why living creatures, including people, age and eventually die. "In the course of these debates, a number of scientists have rallied around a set of ideas called the free radical theory of aging: loosely, the belief that damage by reactive oxygen species [free radicals] is critical in determining life span," reports leading free radical researcher Dr. Bruce Ames from the University of California, Berkeley.

Free radicals are formed in the body as a by-product of the necessary actions of breathing oxygen and burning food for energy. Youth-sapping free radicals are also lurking in air pollution, tobacco smoke, ultraviolet (UV) sun rays, and rancid fats.

Casting free radicals as the villains of the aging process naturally positions antioxidants as the anti-aging heroes. Antioxidants disarm dangerous free radicals before they have a chance to damage proteins, fats, and the genetic material of cells—damage that ultimately leads to aging and death. Although antioxidant nutrients can't stop the hands of time, they may be able to slow down those hands. And naturally, green tea is an especially abundant source of antioxidants.

Linking Tea to a Healthful Lifestyle

A debate is brewing among some researchers over the question of whether tea drinking per se reduces the risk of disease, or the reduction results from other healthful habits practiced by tea drinkers. In other words, it has been suggested that tea merely appears to improve health because tea drinkers happen to be healthier people for other reasons. The leaders of this camp are the authors of a 1996 Dutch study comparing volume of black tea intake with incidence of cancers of the stomach, colon and rectum, lung, and breast. They reported in the *Journal of the National Cancer Institute* that frequent tea imbibers were less likely to develop stomach or lung cancer during the four-year study; however, they attributed this lower cancer risk to the tea drinkers' eating more fruits and vegetables and smoking less. Other researchers questioned this conjecture in a letter to the journal by writing "it is not valid to discount the effects of tea in cancer prevention."[4]

But is all of this debate merely a tempest in a teapot? Tea drinkers do seem, overall, to eat a more healthful diet and lead a more healthful lifestyle, but that should not overshadow the disease-preventing abilities of green tea. Dr. Wei Zheng from the University of Minnesota, who reported his study of tea drinking and cancer risk in 35,000 Iowa women, also noted in his study that tea drinkers ate more fruits and vegetables than non–tea drinkers. However, this did not interfere with his conclusion that the risk for cancer of any site was 10 percent lower among those drinking two or more cups of tea daily.[5]

Another group of researchers questioned whether the results of their study were affected by the healthful diets common to tea drinkers. After examining the health and diet of 1,306 retiring government officials, researchers from the National Defense Medical College in Japan determined that cholesterol levels dropped as tea consumption rose. The researchers asked "whether the relation between green tea and [total cholesterol] was ascribed to other dietary factors. As anticipated, men who consumed greater amounts of green tea tended to adhere to a traditional Japanese diet." Could the lower fat content of the Japanese diet be the true cause of the lower cholesterol levels? After considering this possibility and conducting a statistical analysis regarding this question, the researchers concluded that the green tea was indeed the cause of the lower cholesterol levels.[6]

Coffee is associated with higher cholesterol levels, and since both coffee and tea contain caffeine (although caffeine levels in tea are much lower), some scientists postulated that tea might actually cause cholesterol levels to increase. Just the opposite was found to be true when this issue was investigated; tea (despite its caffeine content) lowers cholesterol levels. An Israeli study that documented a cholesterol-lowering effect for tea also noted that tea drinkers are much less likely to be heavy smokers or alcohol drinkers. Just the opposite is true for coffee drinkers. It would probably be a good idea for coffee drinkers to trade in their cup of coffee for a cup of tea and adopt the other healthful habits of tea drinkers, as well.[7]

A Dutch study indicated that drinking tea is inversely related to smoking cigarettes and eating a fatty diet, but directly related to eating a diet high in vitamin C, vitamin E, beta-carotene, and fiber. And Norwegian investigators found that habitual tea drinkers are among the most likely to use dietary supplements such as vitamins or fish oil.[8]

The healthful habits of tea drinkers that had been revealed incidentally in studies focused on other issues were interesting enough to prompt Dr. Bernhard Schwarz from the University of Vienna, Austria, to undertake a direct comparison of the lifestyles of tea and coffee drinkers. After enrolling 2,400 men and women in the study, he conducted interviews to determine several lifestyle parameters, including smoking, drinking, nutrition, and physical activity. The results were very revealing. The tea drinkers were less likely to eat high-fat dinners, but more likely to consume fish, salads, potatoes, vegetables, and fruits than coffee drinkers. Also, cigarette smokers were more likely to be coffee drinkers, not tea drinkers. The use of tea was associated with an active lifestyle. Tea drinkers more often reported being physically active. Overall, regular coffee intake was associated with negative health behaviors, while drinking tea was linked to a health-conscious, illness-preventive lifestyle.[9]

Becoming "Immune to Aging"

The overall health-promoting effect of polyphenols may account for green tea's role in promoting longevity, particularly since these polyphenols help the immune system function more effectively. Infectious diseases are not a concern of the past. Although vaccines, antibiotics, and other infection-fighting medications have been developed, infections continue to plague mankind. From influenza to HIV, there are some scary bugs out there, and the situation is getting worse, not better. Among the causes of the worsening situation are lifestyles that put people at higher risk of infection, noncompliance with use of prescribed antibiotics, and the emergence of microorganisms that are resistant to antibiotics. Mutations due to the inappropriate and insufficient use of antibiotics is the root cause of this. This naturally raises the question of whether antioxidants and other antimutagenic agents have the capacity of retarding resistance development by pathogens. Encouragingly, there is gathering evidence that this promising hypothesis is true and consumption of green tea and the antioxidant catechins in it appears to be helpful.[10]

Your immune system response, or lack thereof, determines whether you will succumb to the myriad bacteria, viruses, fungi, and other microorganisms you encounter every day or will brush them off and maintain good health. The immune system is an intricate network of specialized tissues, organs, cells, and chemicals whose job descriptions are plain: Seek out and destroy foreign invaders and cancerous cells before they cause illness or death. The lymph nodes, spleen, bone marrow, thymus gland, and tonsils all play a role, as do lymphocytes (specialized white blood cells), antibodies, and interferon.

There are two types of immunity: innate and adaptive. Innate immunity is present at birth and forms the first line of defense against microorganisms. For example, your skin, mucus secretions, and acidity in your stomach act as barriers to keep unwanted germs away from more vulnerable tissues. The second line of defense—called adaptive immunity—is acquired later in life, for example after an immunization or after the body has successfully fought off an infection. The adaptive immune system retains a memory of all the invaders it has ever faced and mobilizes quickly to deal with subsequent exposures. This is why people usually get the measles only once, although they may be exposed to the disease time and again.

Surprisingly, the biggest challenge facing the immune system is poor nutrition. The availability of important nutrients can have a great impact on the course of an infectious disease. Adequate intake of several vitamins, minerals, and herbs enhances the immune system and reduces the risk of developing infection or disease.

The immune system is suppressed during times of stress. Optimal nutrition helps maintain a strong immune system and combat the harmful effects of stress. Other challenges to a healthy immune system include chronic lack of sleep, overwork, and the aging process. Immunity gradually declines over the years, increasing susceptibility to infection. Fortunately, research shows that supplementing the diet with antioxidants can boost immune function back to its "younger" capacity.[11]

Linking Green Tea and Immunity

Green tea drinkers are less likely to be stricken with diseases caused by microorganisms for two reasons. First, green tea polyphenols boost the body's intrinsic defenses against disease (the immune system). Second, polyphenols interact with many microorganisms in such a way as to lessen their disease-causing potential. Yet another reason for tea's disease prevention powers may be strictly hygienic. Tea is safer to drink than water because it is boiled first, and boiling kills most disease-causing organisms that may have been in the water.

As we mentioned earlier in the chapter, the key actors in the body's immune defense system are specialized white blood cells called lymphocytes, which are manufactured in enormous quantities in bone marrow. Some lymphocytes (called B cells) are released directly into the bloodstream; as they circulate, they monitor the blood for microorganism invaders. Other lymphocytes (called T cells) migrate to the thymus gland where they develop into more specialized cells. The T cells attack germs directly and also respond to cancerous cells within the body. The B cells produce antibodies, which in turn work to neutralize potential infection-causing microorganisms and other foreign agents.

According to microbiologists and immunologists from the Showa University School of Medicine in Tokyo, Japan, in the research they conducted on animals "EGCG showed strong immunoenhancement of B-cells." EGCG was the most effective of the catechins in enhancing B cell activity, although ECG also showed some effectiveness. The researchers also noted that catechins boosted activation of macrophages (cells that consume germs), T cells, and natural killer cells (activated white cells that go on "seek-and-destroy" missions against invasive cells).[12]

Most blood cells are produced in bone marrow. Immune-compromising abnormalities can develop as a side effect after chemotherapy or radiation therapy for cancer, both of which interfere with the proper function of the bone marrow. In particular, lowered counts of white blood cells are a common adverse effect of cancer treatment. Not-yet-published research from several Chinese hospitals working with cancer patients demonstrates that green tea polyphenols can boost white blood cell levels, and may accomplish this even better than the standard medications in use. (See Chapter 5 for a more thorough account of these positive studies.)

Certain medications can interfere with the proper function of the immune system. For example, drugs in the thionamides family are generally the first line treatment for hyperthyroidism, but can occasionally result in a dangerous condition called agranulocytosis, in which white blood cells called granulocytes are destroyed, and the body is left vulnerable to infection. Chinese physicians at the Tien Jing Third Central Hospital provided evidence of another immune-supporting effect of green tea when they found that seventy-two hyperthyroid patients who were given green tea polyphenol supplements daily for eight weeks in addition to their regular treatment regimen maintained higher levels of granulocytes and white blood cells than did seventy-five hyperthyroid patients who received standard blood-improving drugs.

In addition, the component in tea called L-theanine, according to research from Brigham and Women's Hospital and Harvard University, contributes to the immune strengthening effect of tea. Apparently, L-theanine improves the ability of the immune system to fight infection, bacteria, viruses, and fungi. When volunteers drank five cups of black tea daily, levels of interferon (a component of the immune system) went up.[13]

Bacterial Infection

One of the earliest reports regarding the anti-infective capability of tea appeared in the *Tea and Coffee Journal* in 1923; it was an army surgeon's recommendation that soldiers carry tea in their water bottles as a way to prevent typhoid infection in regions where the risk of such infection was high. In retrospect, it seems likely that the reason for this recommendation was to ensure that the men would be drinking water that had been boiled, rather than to provide them with the possible antibiotic properties of tea, since those effects are weak. In a review of the antimicrobial properties of tea, Dr. J. M. T. Hamilton-Miller of the Department of Medical Microbiology at the Royal Free Hospital School of Medicine in London noted that tea extracts have been shown to inhibit the growth and reproduction of many species of bacteria, and outright kill them, especially the kinds that cause diseases of the diarrhea type. Furthermore, the amount of tea extract required to achieve these antibacterial effects is generally equivalent to what a person consumes when drinking tea as a beverage. Research efforts to identify the various species of bacteria that green tea polyphenols inhibit are ongoing; so far, the species identified include *Staphylococcus aureus*, *Staphylococcus epidermidis*, *Salmonella typhi*, *Salmonella typhimurium*, *Salmonella enteritidis*, *Shigella flexneri*,

Shigella dysenteriae, and *Clostridium*.[14] Of course, a person who has already contracted a bacterial infection should resort to the use of antibiotics instead of green tea, because green tea is comparatively feeble in its anti-bacterial potency.

Green tea extracts have also been tested to determine their effectiveness in the prevention of several specific bacterial infections. One of these is whooping cough. Although widespread vaccination has made whooping cough uncommon in the United States, it remains a problem in other parts of the world. Whooping cough, or pertussis as it is also called, is caused by the bacterium *Bordetella pertussis*. Japanese researchers have determined that EGCG in green tea and theaflavin in black tea "might act as prophylactic agents against pertussis infection." This prophylactic effect is apparently accomplished through several independent mechanisms, including inhibiting the bacteria from adhering to cells in the body and preventing the pertussis toxin from damaging white blood cells. This group of researchers also found that green and black tea can be used prophylactically against pneumonia infection.[15]

Cholera is an acute infectious disease of the small intestine caused by the bacterium *Vibrio cholerae*; it is characterized by profuse watery diarrhea, vomiting, muscle cramps, severe dehydration, and depletion of electrolytes, and it may lead rapidly to death. Japanese researchers, supported by the Japanese Cholera Panel of the United States–Japan Cooperative Medical Science Program, took a closer look at the bacteria-fighting effects of green tea extract in experiments conducted on animals. They reported that "tea catechins inhibit the activity of cholera toxin, and protect against cholera infection." Furthermore, they recommended that physicians consider adding polyphenols to the therapies currently used in the treatment of cholera patients to hasten their recovery.[16]

Green tea polyphenols have also been shown, in laboratory experiments and trials conducted on animal and human subjects, to inhibit the growth of *Streptococcus mutans,* the bacterium responsible for dental plaque and cavities. (Refer to Chapter 10 for further information on this topic.)

The polyphenols in tea extracts inhibit the growth of both major classes of bacteria: Gram-positive and Gram-negative. These classes, which differ in the structure and composition of the bacterial cell membrane, are classified by the colors they retain when treated with a sequence of dyes in a laboratory procedure developed by Hans C. J. Gram, a Danish physician. To determine how tea polyphenols act as antibacterial agents, Japanese scientists from Tokai University School of Medicine studied the effects of polyphenols on *Escherichia coli* (Gram-negative) and *Staphylococcus aureus* (Gram-positive) bacteria. Of the various polyphenols tested, EGCG was by far the most effective antibacterial agent; it accomplished its antibacterial action by damaging the cell membrane of the bacteria. Although both types of bacteria were susceptible to the tea polyphenols, growth inhibition was more pronounced in the Gram-positive bacteria. The researchers attributed the greater resistance of Gram-negative bacteria to the stronger penetration barrier of the outer membrane of this class of bacteria.[17]

Viral Infection

Scientific confirmation of the antiviral capabilities of tea arrived as early as 1978, when a team from the Bureau of Microbial Hazards in Ottawa, Canada, looked for antiviral agents among nineteen different beverages. The virus that causes polio was used as a representative virus. Tea, grape juice, and apple juice showed the most potent virus-inactivation ability, with less than one percent of the viruses surviving in these beverages. The researchers suggested that flavonoids in these beverages bond with viruses to form noninfectious complexes. Researchers in Japan agree that tea, and EGCG in particular, achieves antiviral effects by interfering with the ability of viruses to adhere to cells.[18]

The influenza virus is also rendered inactive by green tea's polyphenols. Researchers at the National Institute of Health, Tokyo, Japan, discovered that EGCG binds with the flu virus, thereby preventing it from causing an infection. This is a very promising discovery, since influenza causes many deaths throughout the world. A study of mice demonstrated the anti-influenza action of polyphenols in animals. When one group of mice was infected with the influenza virus, all died within ten days. However, when a second group of mice was given polyphenols right after being exposed to the virus, all of the mice survived.[19]

It turns out that even gargling with green tea might help you out during flu season. A study based in Japan, where gargling is viewed by many to be a healthy wintertime habit, had 124 elderly adults gargle with either a green tea solution or plain water three times a day through-out the three months of flu season. Only 1.3% of the green tea group came down with influenza infection, while 10% in the plain water group ended up with the flu.[20]

Perhaps the most exciting research about green tea and viruses has to do with the human immunodeficiency virus (HIV), the virus that causes AIDS.[21] Despite occasional progress and breakthroughs, AIDS research-ers remain frustrated in their search for a way to prevent infection with HIV. EGCG has been reported to inhibit the action of an enzyme called reverse transcriptase (RT), which is essential for the reproduction of HIV. This is the same enzyme that the well-known drug AZT inhib-its. The problem with most agents that inhibit the action of RT is that resistance develops so easily and the RT inhibitors are also very toxic, so that replication of the body's DNA can also be inhibited, leading to many undesirable side effects. EGCG has some potential in preventing AIDS, since it inhibits viral replication at a level five times lower than that at which normal cells are affected. Further research is warranted in this area to confirm these results in human subjects.[22] EGCG may play a role in protecting against acquiring AIDS, but it is unlikely to be useful after AIDS is acquired. It is no substitute for taking precautions to avoid exposure to the virus, or AZT or protease inhibitors and other powerful drugs.

The human papillomavirus (HPV) is a very common sexually trans-mitted infection. More than 6 million new cases are contracted every year in the United States. There are more than 100 different types of HPV; while the majority of these are harmless, others are not. This virus can lead to the development of genital warts, although many people infected with HPV have no outward signs or symptoms. Some types of HPV can lead to cervical cancer. Recently, vaccines to protect against HPV have been developed, although these vaccines do not protect against all the types of HPV.

Genital warts can be removed by several methods, including freezing (cryosurgery). A new (and nonpainful) treatment for genital warts has been developed based on a green tea extract. This green tea ointment, called Polyphenon E, has been shown in clinical trials to remove external genital warts. Polyphenon E ointment is thought to work by interfering with the growth of HPV, as well as by stimulating the immune system.

Keeping the Liver Healthy

The liver is a very important organ that performs thousands of vital chemical and metabolic functions, including the storage of fat-soluble vitamins, iron, and glycogen (a form of carbohydrate) for when the body needs these nutrients at a later date. In addition, it makes cholesterol and amino acids, removes wastes from the blood, detoxifies alcohol and other toxins, and breaks down many medications.

Unlike most other organs, the liver can regenerate itself. Even so, it can be damaged severely by disease or toxins beyond the point of repair. Alcohol is the leading cause of liver disease, often leading to the liver disease cirrhosis. The scarring in the liver caused by cirrhosis is irreversible. As with all liver problems, stopping drinking alcohol is essential to preventing further damage. After cirrhosis, hepatitis is the next most common liver disease. There are many different types of hepatitis, and unfortunately there are not a lot of conventional treatment options for any of them, aside from rest and avoidance of alcohol.

Anyone with a liver disease should choose a diet that is the least burdensome to the liver. This means absolutely no alcohol, minimizing fatty foods, and eating only small amounts of protein. Proteins from plant sources, such as grains and legumes, are easier for the liver to handle than animal source proteins. A low-salt diet and plenty of fluids are also important.

Every breath we take, every glass of water we drink, and every bite of food we eat is a potential source of toxins. Reducing your exposure to toxins is an important way to protect the body, but many times toxins are simply unavoidable; they are in air pollution, tobacco smoke, pesticide residue, and some artificial flavors and colorings. The liver can be hit especially hard by toxins, since the job of the liver is to clear the blood of poisonous substances before they have a chance to reach other parts of the body. Tea polyphenols support the liver's enzyme detoxification system, which eliminates free radicals and toxins from the body.

The liver is without a doubt the biggest gun in the body's detoxification arsenal. The liver is the largest internal organ, weighing in at about three pounds. It is red-brown in color, roughly coneshaped, and seated in the upper right corner of the abdominal cavity. The liver performs several important functions for the body, such as regulating levels of amino acids in the blood and producing important proteins for blood plasma. The liver is so resilient that it will continue to perform its vital functions even when as much as three-quarters of it has been destroyed or removed.

However, the liver's most valuable function in our increasingly polluted world may be clearing the blood of drugs and poisonous substances that would otherwise accumulate in the bloodstream and other areas of the body. The liver achieves the cleansing action by absorbing toxic substances from the bloodstream and, with the help of enzymes, altering their chemical structure to make them water-soluble. The poisons can then be excreted from the body in the bile or the urine. The bile is dumped into the intestine, where some is taken up again and recycled, and some is excreted in the feces.

Catechins can help the liver's enzyme systems function more effectively and protect the liver itself from the toxins it is detoxifying. Other research shows that green tea, in animals, prevents liver injuries caused by viral infections. When Japanese epidemiologists surveyed the diets and tracked the liver health of 1,371 adult men, they discovered that "increased consumption of green tea, especially more than ten cups a day, was related to decreased concentrations of hepatological markers" that would indicate cell damage to the liver.[23]

Although the general function of the liver is to protect the body, it can cause harm by activating carcinogens through the cytochrome P450 enzyme system in the liver. Again, green tea comes to the rescue. Green tea extracts minimize the effect of carcinogens by inhibiting the P450 enzymes.[24]

Green tea also shows a strong effect in preventing poisoning by aflatoxin. Aflatoxin is a group of toxins produced by certain *Aspergillus* molds that can contaminate peanuts, other nuts, grains, and corn stored in warm, humid environments. After being consumed in the contaminated food, these toxins are oxidized in the liver, which can cause specific genetic mutations that are highly correlated to the risk of liver cancer. In fact, in areas of the world with prevalent aflatoxin contamination, up to half of the liver tumors can be traced back to this toxin.

Of course, you should avoid aflatoxin-contaminated foods (such as old or damaged peanuts), but if aflatoxin exposure does occur, green tea can minimize the damage. Green tea extract protects the genetic material from aflatoxin damage by inhibiting oxidation of aflatoxin in the liver.[25]

Supporting Health in Diabetes

Diabetes, although found around the globe, is particularly prevalent in the United States. By some estimates, as many as half of all the world's diabetics live in the United States. Our "affluent" diet and lifestyle is often to blame. Diabetes has become so common that complications from diabetes rank as the sixth leading cause of death among Americans.

Insulin, a hormone produced by the pancreas, is made in response to the level of glucose (sugar) in the bloodstream. Insulin serves two purposes: It lowers blood sugar levels and increases the availability of sugar for normal cell functioning. Normally, after a meal, complex carbohydrates are digested and absorbed from the intestine into the bloodstream in the form of glucose and other simple sugars. This resulting rise in blood sugar causes the pancreas to secrete insulin, which encourages the transportation of sugar from the blood into the cells. As blood sugar levels fall, blood insulin levels return to the pre-meal state.

Things happen differently for diabetics. Either the pancreas secretes little or no insulin in response to the rise in blood sugar after a meal or the pancreas secretes a normal amount of insulin but the cells do not respond to the hormone. In either case, the result is that blood sugar levels remain high; sugar spills into the urine, and many complications can develop in the body from the abnormal blood sugar levels.

There are two types of diabetes. The first is called type 1, insulin-dependent, or juvenile-onset diabetes. It usually begins in childhood and develops very quickly. Type 1 diabetics, who account for only ten percent of the diabetes population, usually have reduced numbers of active beta cells in the pancreas; those are the cells responsible for the production and secretion of insulin. The person with type 1 diabetes must inject insulin and balance the entry of insulin into the blood with food intake to maintain normal use of sugar.

The other 90 percent of diabetics are called type 2, non-insulin-dependent, or adult-onset diabetics. Type 2 diabetes usually begins in the adult years and progresses more slowly. Although genetic factors contribute to a person's risk for developing type 2 diabetes, lifestyle factors, such as being overweight, consuming a poor diet, and lack of exercise are also important. Type 2 diabetics often secrete adequate amounts of insulin, but their cells are not sufficiently sensitive to the hormone.

Although it is not the first-line treatment for diabetes, green tea may provide some benefits to the diabetic beyond those brought by diet and drugs. Epicatechin has been shown to bring high blood sugar levels in diabetic animals back down to normal values. In addition, the beta cells of these animals, which were previously found to be inactive, were regenerated with the polyphenol and regained their proper function. Other researchers report that epicatechin, besides promoting the secretion of insulin, also acts with insulin-like properties in the body. In all, the animal research suggests that tea has a preventive effect on diabetes. There is a word of caution from the body of literature: One isolated study suggests that children who regularly consume tea have an increased risk of type 1 diabetes.[26]

In a very large study including more than 17,000 people spread across twenty-five different communities in Japan, researchers looked into any connections between beverage choices and risk of developing diabetes.[27] After following their health for five years, researchers learned that drinking green tea had an inverse relationship to the risk of developing diabetes. There was no association for black or oolong teas. At this point, the research points to a protective role of green tea against diabetes.

Keeping the Kidneys in Good Health

The kidneys filter out and remove waste products from the blood, help maintain the normal range of nutrients in the blood, and regulate the body's pH level (acid-base balance). Kidney disorders range in severity from temporary loss of appetite to tissue deterioration and death. Chronic renal failure—the condition in which the kidneys are unable to perform their task of filtering waste out of the blood—can result from several causes, including infection, injury, diabetic complication, or cancer. However, animal-based research suggests that green tea extract improves kidney function in cases of chronic renal failure, even in the face of free radical overload. Studies of specialized kidney cells grown in the laboratory indicate that green tea retards the progression of chronic renal failure. Additionally, the abnormal growth of certain kidney cells is quelled, particularly in cases of diabetes-related kidney failure.[28]

Drinking more fluids in general is recommended to anyone who has had a kidney stone in order to reduce the chances of getting another one. When a group of 81,093 women were tracked for eight years, researchers found that what beverage the women drank regularly could make a big difference in terms of the development of kidney stones. For every 8-ounce cup of tea consumed each day, the risk of developing kidney stones was reduced by 8 percent. A similar study with 45,289 men showed a similar relationship, with each cup of tea resulting in a 14 percent lower risk of stone development.[29]

Chinese physicians have taken an interest in the ability of green tea extract to assist with the health problems associated with chronic renal failure. After treating twenty-five patients with this condition, physicians at the First People's Hospital of Xiao Shan City in the Zhe Jiang Province of China reported very promising results. All of these patients, who had a variety of diseases responsible for their kidney failure, including diabetes, hypertensive renal disease, and infections, received the standard treatment protocol (low salt, high-quality protein diet) while half were also given dietary supplements of green tea polyphenols. The polyphenol group showed significant improvements in their condition, as evidenced by improved blood and urine profiles and less puffiness, lumbago, fatigue, and dizziness.[30] One can infer from this that, short of acute renal failure, green tea can be a useful supplement to drug therapy.

Long Sai Hospital physicians in Ning Bo, China, reported similarly positive results from treating sixty cases of chronic renal insufficiency. Again, half of the patients received the usual care, and the other half received green tea polyphenol supplements in addition to the standard treatment. Kidney function in the green tea group was significantly improved after one and two months of supplementation. The physicians speculated that the ability of green tea to disarm free radicals played a role in the beneficial effects for kidney patients.[31]

Keeping the Mind Sharp

Most people, as they age, experience some decline in memory, learning ability, and concentration. By some estimates, the average person's cognitive abilities can decline by as much as half with the passage of time. Part of the underlying cause is the fact that over time the number of brain cells damaged by free radicals increases until it manifests itself in a discernible decline of mental function. Antioxidants—including EGCG—are a great way to protect mental acuity that is threatened by the mounting effects of free radical attacks. Researchers at the Science University of Tokyo, Japan, have concluded that "the effect of tea catechins in promoting neurons of normal learning ability . . . may be related to their ability to scavenge active oxygen species. . . . [As a result of this ability, they] might become useful for protecting humans from senile disorders such as dementia."[32]

The mental protection hypothesized by the aforementioned study was demonstrated in forty-six cases of cerebrovascular disease (including twenty-two patients with dementia) studied by physicians at the Beijing Tian Tan Affiliated Hospital of Capital Medical University in China. All of these patients, who had significant cognitive impairments, were given green tea polyphenol supplements daily for one month; no other brain-function-improving drugs were given for the duration of the study. An impressive 91 percent of the dementia patients and 60 percent of the patients with verbal disorders showed significant improvement. The physicians noted that the earlier in the course of the disease's progression the polyphenols were given, the better the effect.

The caffeine content of green tea may also contribute to the beverage's support of clear thinking. Scientific studies show that caffeine (from any source) enhances cognitive performance, particularly for reaction time, spatial relationships, and certain aspects of memory. Caffeine also staves off boredom and mental fatigue. Researchers have found that caffeine consumption increases a subject's feeling of well-being, energy level, and motivation to work.

Alzheimer's Disease

Alzheimer's disease is a medical mystery: Its cause is unknown, it is difficult to diagnose, and there is no cure. Over the past several decades, the scientific community has been working hard to unravel this puzzling disease. And just over the past few years, Alzheimer's disease has finally begun to give up some of its secrets.

Four and a half million Americans are estimated to be afflicted with Alzheimer's disease, with perhaps the most well-known victim being former president Ronald Reagan. Although the death toll of Alzheimer's is significant, the biggest tragedy is the loss of memory, reasoning power, and ability to carry out daily functions that Alzheimer's disease victims suffer in the years and sometimes decades before death.

The condition of dementia is common in older adults, and is characterized by a decline in intellectual and social abilities. Approximately half of the cases of dementia in the elderly are accounted for by Alzheimer's disease.

Back in 1907, Alois Alzheimer identified characteristic changes in the brain cells of individuals with the disease that now bears his name. Although this discovery of structural changes to the brain is interesting, it is not useful for diagnostic purposes, since it would require a brain biopsy. Furthermore, there is a controversy as to whether these structural changes are causes, results, or merely events occurring at the same time as Alzheimer's disease. Instead of relying on these physical signs, doctors rely on tracking the symptoms of an individual.

The hallmark symptoms of Alzheimer's disease are:

- the gradual loss of memory for recent events
- inability to learn new information
- mental confusion
- personality changes
- behavior changes, such as irritability, anxiety, and/or depression

Symptoms typical to Alzheimer's disease, such as memory loss and mental confusion, can be caused by many other conditions. It is crucial to rule out these other conditions before diagnosing Alzheimer's. For instance, vitamin B_{12} deficiencies are very common in the elderly and can cause similar cognitive changes as seen in Alzheimer's disease. Unlike Alzheimer's disease, a vitamin B_{12} deficiency is easily treated. Therefore it is important that a patient receives a thorough diagnosis and not simply be assumed to have Alzheimer's without exploring other possible causes for their symptoms.

Free radicals, the infamous culprits underlying most degenerative diseases, are also thought to play a role in Alzheimer's disease. Free radicals may set the stage for Alzheimer's by damaging brain cells. Whenever free radicals are thought to instigate a disease, it makes sense to consider the benefits of antioxidants—which can be thought of as free radical antidotes.

Naturally, green tea provides copious amounts of antioxidants. But that may not be the only way that green tea delays the onset of this disease. Research shows that both green and black teas block certain brain enzymes that are linked to the development of Alzheimer's.[33] Laboratory tests indicate that tea inhibits activity of brain chemicals that could otherwise contribute to the creation of plaques and tangles in the brain, which are problems seen in Alzheimer's. Green tea was more powerful than black tea in this regard. Of course, tea is not an Alzheimer's cure, but it certainly might provide a bit of insurance against the development of this disease at an early age.

In addition, there are some early indications that green tea could also provide some neuroprotection against Parkinson's disease, which is another brain condition.[34]

Stress and Anxiety

The amino acid L-theanine, found almost exclusively in the tea plant, not only contributes to the unique taste of tea, but it also counteracts some of the stimulant effects of caffeine and leads to a relaxed state.

L-theanine is unique as an amino acid, since it is one of the few amino acids to penetrate readily into the brain, where it partly counteracts the stimulation of caffeine and interacts with brain receptors that are associated with relaxation.[35] Certain neurotransmitters (namely serotonin and dopamine) are altered after ingesting L-theanine, and it's these changes in the brain that trigger relaxation without a loss of clear thinking. In one study of university students, taking 200 milligrams of L-theanine eased anxiety and increased alpha brain wave activity after forty minutes; alpha brain waves are the type associated with relaxation.[36]

Arthritis and Inflammatory Diseases

Green tea is now known to have several anti-inflammatory effects. This opens the door to research in the area of arthritis, gout, and other inflammatory conditions. Inflammation is closely associated with the effects of reactive oxygen species, so an effect of green tea antioxidants is logical. There are no studies with humans demonstrating arthritis relief from drinking tea as yet, but it is interesting to note that this is an area that researchers have their eye on.

Sickle Cell Anemia

Sickle cell anemia affects millions of people and is an inherited (genetic) disorder in which the body makes abnormally shaped red blood cells due to a mutation that leads to substitution of a single amino acid for the normal amino acid in one of the subunits of hemoglobin. Red blood cells should be smooth and circular, but in sickle cell disease, they are crescent shaped (like a sickle). This abnormal shape is not able to flow easily through the blood vessels, and because they are also hard and sticky, they tend to get stuck and block the flow of blood to the limbs and organs. The end result can be pain, organ damage, and anemia (since the altered hemoglobin is shorter lived than normal hemoglobin). There are some treatments but no cure for sickle cell. The comparative prevalence of sickle cell trait in certain regions of the earth comes from the resistance of sufferers to developing malaria. The choice between malaria and sickle cell anemia is a cruel one!

The extra "dense" blood cells of sickle cell anemia are generally the source of painful episodes with this disease. Currently, there is some evidence that green tea extract can greatly reduce (actually cut in half) the formation of these dense cells.[37]

Sensible lifestyle choices, of course, play a crucial role in a long, healthy life; but the effects of nutrition should not be underestimated. A healthy diet combined with some superstar nutrients can be a great way to boost longevity and extend health span. By reducing the likelihood that a person will die prematurely from heart disease or cancer, green tea goes a long way toward extending longevity. However, maintaining a high quality of life throughout the span of life is even more desirable than simply living longer, and green tea, as we have seen, can help maintain good health. Green tea keeps the immune system running smoothly to help prevent infections, aids the body's detoxification system, and may even keep the mind sharp and stress levels in check. All of those functions are important for maintaining the highest level of wellness throughout the life span. Of course, there is no guarantee that drinking green tea will prolong your life, but it is certainly a pleasurable active step that may, in fact, contribute to a healthier life.

chapter eight

A "Nice Cup of Tea" for Digestion

The enjoyment of a good meal is one of life's pleasures. When the gut works right, as with most organs, we don't notice it. Unfortunately, trouble can start brewing as soon as a mouthful of your favorite dish is swallowed. Faulty digestion causes a lot of unnecessary discomfort due to heartburn, bloating, gas, and sour stomach. Digestion problems also contribute to many gastrointestinal and related health problems, such as diarrhea, peptic ulcer, and Crohn's disease.

Throughout history, people of many cultures have enjoyed a cup of tea with or after their meals, and the practice continues in modern times. Of course, the primary inspiration for this practice is the pleasing taste of tea beverages, but the tea habit also has beneficial effects on the digestive process. Its benefits include improved digestion, decreased risk of ulcers, inflammatory bowel disease relief, and assistance in maintaining a healthy weight.

The Digestive Tract

The digestive system is composed of several parts that all work in concert to digest and absorb food. The digestive system can be thought of as a tube approximately sixteen and one-half feet long extending from the mouth to the anus. It includes the esophagus, stomach, small intestine, pancreas, gallbladder, liver, and large intestine. Most of the mechanical

The Digestive Tract

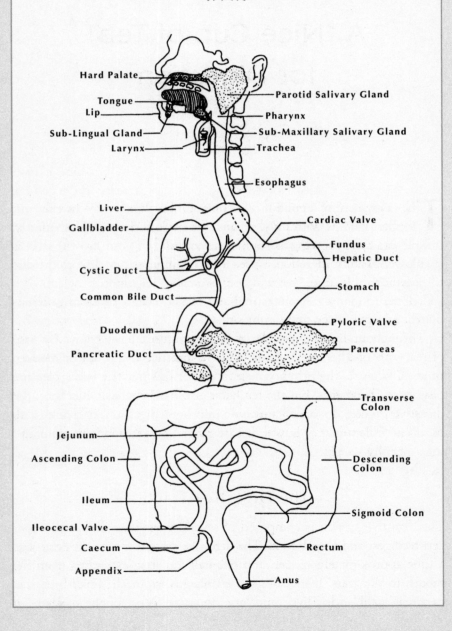

Hard Palate

Tongue
Lip
Sub-Lingual Gland
Larynx

Parotid Salivary Gland
Pharynx
Sub-Maxillary Salivary Gland
Trachea

Esophagus

Liver
Gallbladder

Cardiac Valve

Fundus
Hepatic Duct

Cystic Duct

Common Bile Duct

Stomach

Duodenum

Pyloric Valve

Pancreatic Duct

Pancreas

Transverse Colon

Jejunum

Ascending Colon

Descending Colon

Ileum

Ileocecal Valve

Sigmoid Colon

Caecum

Rectum

Appendix

Anus

and chemical breakdown of food to make it absorbable occurs in gastrointestinal tract, which consists of the stomach (*gaster* in Greek) and the intestine.

The whole digestive system starts to work as soon as a bite of food enters the mouth. The process of chewing mashes the food into smaller, more manageable pieces. Meanwhile, an enzyme called amylase, contained in saliva, begins the chemical breakdown of carbohydrates into simple sugars. If you chew a piece of bread or other starchy food long enough, you'll notice a sweet taste when the starch is turned into sugar by the amylase. Next, the food is swallowed; that is, it travels down the throat and the esophagus, a tube that connects the throat to the stomach. A series of wave-like contractions keeps the food moving down to the stomach.

In the stomach, powerful muscles churn the food, breaking it into smaller and smaller pieces and mixing it with gastric juices produced by the glands lining the stomach. These juices contain pepsin, an enzyme that begins to digest proteins, and hydrochloric acid to acidify the food. Only alcohol, simple sugars, and some medications are actually absorbed from the stomach. Continued wave-like contractions move the food from the stomach through the rest of the gastrointestinal tract.

The next stop is the small intestine, where the majority of nutrient absorption takes place. The food is further prepared for absorption by digestive enzymes from the pancreas and intestinal lining and by bile from the gallbladder and liver. Billions of specialized cells line the small intestine and absorb the end-products of digestion, including amino acids from protein, sugar from carbohydrates, fatty acids from fats, and cholesterol, vitamins, and minerals. What's left over—water, undigested fibers, some minerals, bile, and waste products—is shuttled to the large intestine. Most of the water and bile acids are reabsorbed, and the rest of the large intestine's contents are excreted from the body.

Green Tea as a Digestive Aid

Green tea goes through the digestive process itself, of course; along the way, it exerts certain positive effects on the process. To confirm that the polyphenols in green tea are absorbed from the gastrointestinal tract, a group of researchers from the Department of Nutritional Science and

Dietetics at the University of Nebraska developed a fifty-six-day study using ten healthy adults in a laboratory atmosphere. During four separate fourteen-day periods, all the adults ate a controlled diet; in each period, they drank a different beverage at each of their three meals: green tea, regular black tea, decaffeinated black tea, or beverages other than tea. Analyses of samples of the subjects' blood, urine, and feces showed detectable levels of polyphenols in all of the dietary periods that included tea, but green tea led to the highest levels. Clearly, tea polyphenols—and particularly those from green tea—are absorbed by the gastrointestinal tract and make their way throughout the body.[1]

Polyphenols from green tea affect carbohydrate metabolism in several ways. First, polyphenols inhibit the function of amylase, the enzyme in saliva that starts the digestive process of carbohydrates. This diminishes the absorption of glucose derived from complex carbohydrates. Second, polyphenols inhibit the enzymes sucrase and glucosidase, which are necessary for carbohydrate digestion in the small intestine. Third, green tea extracts alter the transport mechanism used to bring glucose across the intestinal barrier. The end result is reduced absorption of carbohydrates and lower blood glucose levels, which may be beneficial in cases of diabetes or obesity.[2]

Green tea is also a source of vitamins. Aside from the polyphenols, vitamin C is probably the most prevalent nutrient in green tea. A gram of green tea provides about two milligrams of vitamin C. Vitamin C levels in black tea are much lower, since much of this vitamin is lost during the oxidation process. Other vitamins found in varying amounts in tea are vitamin B_2, vitamin D, vitamin K, and the carotenoids (a family of fat-soluble pigments). The minerals present in green tea include chromium, calcium, magnesium, manganese, iron, copper, zinc, molybdenum, selenium, sodium, phosphorus, strontium, cobalt, nickel, and potassium. Tea, and green tea in particular, is also an impressive source of fluoride—the mineral well known for fighting cavities. The water used in brewing tea as a beverage also contributes to its mineral content.

Some health-care providers warn people against drinking tea if they are taking iron supplements (in the non-hemic ferrous salt form), since early research suggested that the tea could interfere with the absorption of iron, and possibly other minerals. But this concern appears to be unfounded. In a study of four elderly patients with iron-deficiency anemia and eleven healthy older adults, supplements of iron increased blood levels of iron equally well in both anemic and non-anemic people, whether they drank green tea or did not.[3] Another study, this one involving anemic pregnant women taking iron, reports that the anemia was actually cured in slightly more of the green tea drinkers than in the green-tea abstainers. It would seem that not only does green tea *not* interfere with iron absorption, but that the opposite may be true: green tea may help resolve iron-deficiency states.[4] And there is certainly no reason for healthy people who have no risk factors for anemia to restrict their tea consumption.

Some experts also expressed concern that certain teas had been found to contain high levels of aluminum, which could increase the risk of certain bone and brain disorders. Fortunately, when later researchers investigated this issue, they discovered that the aluminum in tea is present in a complex form that is less absorbable than the ionic form of aluminum and has much less potential to exert an adverse effect on health. Experiments on animals and people confirmed this hypothesis, since the frequent consumption of green tea did not contribute significantly to the body's aluminum burden, nor did aluminum accumulate in the bones. It would seem that the "aluminum issue" is not a true health concern in the case of tea.[5]

Green tea contains several common amino acids, as well as an amino acid that is unique to it: theanine. Theanine accounts for about half of the total of amino acids in green tea, and the amount of theanine is said to correlate with the quality of the final tea product. And, as was discussed earlier in this book, L-theanine appears to have numerous health benefits, including easing anxiety, reducing the risk of cardiovascular disease, and fighting cancer.

Green tea protects the digestive tract from carcinogens that could otherwise harm the stomach, intestine, or colon and could even influence cancer development throughout the body. Among these harmful carcinogens is a class of mutagens derived by metabolic oxidation of certain heterocyclic amines (HCA). These potentially harmful HCAs are formed during the cooking, especially frying, of meats and fish and enter the digestive tract when the food is eaten. They are believed to be a major contributor to cancer. Dr. John H. Weisburger from the American Health Foundation noted in a report of his research that "use of polyphenols may be a practical means of blocking the formation of HCAs during cooking," but the green tea must be added to the meat or fish dish during cooking.[6] How green tea affects the taste of a steak has not been reported. Researchers at the British Columbia Cancer Research Center in Vancouver, British Columbia, investigated the effects of green tea on nitrosamination, a cancer-promoting process. They reported that "the simultaneous intake of teas with food products that are being nitrosated within the stomach of human subjects should exert a protective, beneficial effect."[7]

More than four hundred different species of bacteria live in the intestinal tract; fortunately less than 1 percent of these bacteria are harmful, but that 1 percent can have a negative effect on health, for example by causing diarrhea or constipation. On the other hand, the beneficial bacteria increase the body's resistance to infection, help maintain bowel regularity, and promote digestion. Maintaining healthy colonies of beneficial bacteria is very important to good digestive health. Green tea promotes a healthy digestive tract by altering the intestinal environment to make it favorable to the growth of the friendly bacteria and less favorable to the growth of undesirable bacteria. If potentially harmful bacteria proliferate unchecked by friendly bacteria, the chances are greater that a species of bacteria will grow to sufficient numbers to influence bowel health—causing either diarrhea or constipation. A study of thirty-seven human volunteers found that green tea increased the regularity of bowel movements. At the beginning of the study, only half of the volunteers reported regular bowel movements, but the number increased to more than 80 percent after twelve weeks of a diet supplemented with green tea polyphenols.[8] Animal studies have shown similar improvements in intestinal digestion after ingesting green tea, indicated by a noticeably reduced odor from the feces.[9]

Indigestion

Every once in a while about half of us suffer from indigestion—an umbrella term to describe symptoms such as heartburn, upset stomach, bloating, gas, and slow digestion—and 25 million Americans face indigestion as a daily part of life. It doesn't have to be this way, since there are many natural remedies for this common condition.

There is often no specific culprit in indigestion. Other times, w... bit of sleuthing, you can determine the cause of your dyspepsia and take steps to remedy the underlying condition. All too often, indigestion is simply the result of eating too much, eating too quickly, or eating while under too much stress.

Avoiding the foods or situations that seem to trigger a bout of indigestion is often the best and simplest way to treat this problem. An indigestion prevention plan should be based on a wholesome, low-fat diet. Fatty foods can lead to indigestion, since they take longer to digest and result in a full, bloated feeling and even pain. Overeating is another red flag; smaller meals at regular intervals are a better choice. If indigestion is a result of a food allergy or intolerance, then avoiding the problem food can be an easy fix.

Alcohol and tobacco can trigger sour stomach. Smokers can help relieve their indigestion by stopping smoking (quitting is, of course, good for overall health) or at least not smoking right before eating.

When and how meals are eaten can be another tie to indigestion. Exercising with a full stomach is a sure way, for many people, to bring on a sour stomach. The digestive system requires a tremendous amount of blood to process food, and putting muscles to work diverts this needed blood. Scheduling exercise before a meal or waiting for an hour helps keep digestion moving properly.

On the other hand, you don't want to completely shut your body down after a meal. Lying down or even slouching after a meal can bring on a bout of heartburn, since these positions increase stomach pressure. A good rule of thumb is to wait two hours after eating before going to bed. In addition, raising the head of the bed by three to six inches can help by using the force of gravity to keep the stomach in place and prevent a reflux of stomach acids.

Green tea (as well as the other varieties of tea) has a long history of use in easing the discomfort of indigestion. It certainly wouldn't hurt to give it a try if your stomach feels unsettled.

Diarrhea

Episodes of loose watery stools that occur three or more times in one day are generally considered to be diarrhea. Abdominal cramps, nausea, vomiting, fever, loss of appetite, and bloody or foul-smelling stools are often present as well. Many serious diseases can cause diarrhea (including infections that continue to rank as a leading killer of Third World children, primarily due to dehydration), but this discussion is limited to the common, run-of-the-mill diarrhea bouts that tend to resolve themselves within forty-eight hours. Diarrhea lasting longer than this will need to be treated by a physician, rather than with at-home remedies.

The most important thing to do for diarrhea is to stay hydrated. Diarrhea causes the body to lose lots of fluids, and this risk of dehydration is the most common medical consequence of ordinary diarrhea. It cannot be emphasized strongly enough: During a boat of diarrhea, drink lots of water or other fluids—which, as you might suspect, can certainly include tea in all its varieties. Tea is very astringent (which lessens intestinal inflammation), and in this way helps during diarrhea.[10] Compounds called tannins account for the astringency of tea; and the longer you brew your cup of tea, the more tannins (and hence anti-diarrheal effect) there will be.

As your diarrhea subsides, you'll want to continue with tea intake, while being gentle to your recovering intestines by eating a simple diet that is easily processed, such as carrot soup, dry cereal, crackers, mashed potatoes, or other foods that seem appetizing during your recovery. For the next day or two, avoid dairy products, high-protein foods, and fatty foods.

Green Tea as an Ulcer Preventive

Ulcers are a common problem, affecting one out of every ten people at some time in their lifetime. The most frequently reported symptom is a burning, aching, or gnawing feeling in the upper abdomen or lower chest. Nausea and vomiting can also occur.

An ulcer is any sore on the body, but when someone says that they have an ulcer, they almost always mean a "peptic" ulcer. Peptic ulcers develop when the mucous membrane lining the stomach or the duodenum is eroded and no longer able to protect the tissue below. An intact mucous lining is essential in protecting us from strong gastric acid and digestive enzymes thus preventing us from digesting our own stomachs. Men are four times more likely than women to have an ulcer.

For many years, stress and spicy foods were thought to be at the of peptic ulcers. Today, both of these things are off the hook (although stress and diet can certainly aggravate an existing ulcer). The real culprit of most ulcers is the bacterium *Helicobacter pylori* (*H. pylori*). The hostile environment of the stomach helps us resist infection by most common bacteria taken in by ingestion of non-sterile food and drink. *H. pylori* is exceptional among bacteria in being able to thrive in stomach fluids. It also, however, erodes the stomach lining in many people. This bacterium was discovered to be present in many ulcer sufferers in 1982. Researchers subsequently found that antibiotics can destroy *H. pylori* and cure peptic ulcers. Other ulcers can be caused by use of nonsteroidal anti-inflammatory agents (NSAIDs), like aspirin and ibuprofen since they interfere with the body's ability to produce the mucous lining of the stomach. These drugs should be avoided by anyone with peptic ulcers. Newer agents like Vioxx and Celebrex are less likely to erode the stomach lining but can cause cardiac complications in some patients.

Infection with *H. pylori* is quite common, with about 20 percent of people under the age of forty and 50 percent of those over the age of sixty having it. Fortunately, just having the bacteria does not mean that an ulcer is inevitable—most infected people, in fact, do not develop ulcers. It is not yet known what other factors cause *H. pylori* to trigger an ulcer. It is known, however, that *H. pylori* is able to weaken the protective mucous membrane that lines the stomach and duodenum, thus allowing the damaging stomach acid and pepsin to reach the sensitive tissue beneath to cause an ulcer. *H. pylori* is also known to increase the risk of stomach cancer in persons ingesting pro-carcinogenic agents.

This comparatively recent discovery has transformed the treatment of ulcers. In healthy people, the linings of the esophagus, stomach, and small intestine act as a barrier to the corrosive chemical nature and enzymes of digestive juices. When a hole or break in this lining occurs, this balance is disturbed and ulcer symptoms occur because of damage to the underlying structures.

A completely bland diet was once de rigueur for anyone with an ulcer, but now that *H. pylori*, as opposed to spicy foods, is known to cause ulcers the thinking on this has changed. Even so, if you notice that certain spicy foods, or any other particular foods, worsen your ulcer, it makes sense to avoid it them. There is some evidence that food allergies might play a role in peptic ulcers. Thus, it might be helpful to determine if food allergies are present and avoid those foods. Salty foods can irritate the stomach, and it would be prudent to restrict the use of salt. Likewise, alcohol and coffee (caffeinated as well as decaf) should also be avoided.

The catechins in tea may help prevent ulcers. In tests conducted on animals, catechins showed an 80-percent success rate in preventing stomach ulcers. In another animal study, normally brewed black tea given to rats inhibited the formation of ulcers, even when the rats consumed aspirin and other medications that can increase the risk of ulcers.[11] While it might not provide complete resolution to the ulcer problem, it certainly seems that green tea might have a role in blocking the H. pylori in ulcers.[12]

Inflammatory Bowel Disease:
Crohn's Disease and Ulcerative Colitis

One million Americans know the pain of inflammatory bowel disease—an umbrella term for Crohn's disease and ulcerative colitis. Both of these cause inflammation of the intestines, but the difference is that ulcerative colitis affects only the colon and rectum, while Crohn's disease—the more serious of the two—involves more extensive areas of the intestines.

These diseases are growing at a rate that has both alarmed and baffled doctors. Crohn's disease, named after the doctor who first identified the disease in the 1930s, doubled in occurrence between then and 1970, and its incidence has subsequently tripled. This sharp increase is particularly vexing since the most common victim is in the prime of his or her life (that is, ages twenty to forty). The hallmark signs of Crohn's are chronic diarrhea, abdominal cramps and pain, a low-grade fever, fatigue, and weight loss. It can seem as though food has turned against you, since the episodes of pain and diarrhea, which can be quite severe and debilitating, generally follow mealtime.

What could be fueling this epidemic? Experts are still unclear about the specifics, but they do know that there is something in our Western lifestyle that must be the culprit since the highest concentration of new cases are in Western countries. What is known is that having a relative with Crohn's disease can put you at ten times greater risk of developing the disease yourself, and if that relative is a sibling, then your risk jumps to thirty times greater than average. Aside from this genetic link, Crohn's disease seems to be triggered by something in the environment (perhaps a bacteria or virus) that sets off an abnormal immune response.

The really bad news is that Crohn's disease has no cure, and the standard treatments can often impair quality of life as much as the disease itself. Drugs such as steroids, aspirin-like medications, and immune suppressants are among the standard arsenal. Almost three-quarters of those with Crohn's end up having surgery to remove inflamed areas of intestine or deal with related complications of the disease. However, even this drastic measure is not a long-term fix since the disease recurs in almost all cases.

Good nutrition and dietary supplements play important roles in Crohn's disease. First, they can prolong periods of remission and, second, they can provide some relief of symptoms during an active episode of the disease. Food allergies appear to be involved with Crohn's disease. Many people report that their disease flares up when certain trigger foods are eaten. Which foods act as triggers is particular to each individual; however, spicy foods, high-fiber foods, milk, and alcohol are common culprits. It's worth the time to sleuth out which foods could be setting you off.

Deficiencies of numerous vitamins and minerals are common in those with Crohn's disease, in large part due to the chronic diarrhea that flushes away nutrients before the body can use them. A multi-vitamin/mineral supplement can provide some measure of protection against deficiencies.

Individuals with inflammatory bowel diseases might be helped by green tea; it helps reduce inflammation associated with these diseases. Green tea helps in another way, too: it helps prevent colon cancer, which is the type of cancer people with inflammatory bowel disease are at high risk of developing. Free radicals are thought to play a role in these diseases—both for initiation and progression—so obviously the powerful antioxidants in green tea fit the bill as a way to counteract this free radical challenge.[13] In addition, green tea can help in these conditions by easing the inflammation that is present. Research has, in fact, shown promise for green tea polyphenols in these conditions.

Green Tea as a Secret Weapon for Weight Loss

Any successful long-term weight reduction results primarily from eating less and expending more calories. A cup of tea (without added sugar or milk) provides only four calories, which certainly makes this beverage acceptable for any weight-loss diet. Weight-loss experts hypothesize that green tea reduces the rate and amount of dietary carbohydrates absorbed, but without putting the body at risk of malnutrition. The polyphenols in green tea influence the action of amylase, the enzyme in saliva that digests carbohydrates, and also influence the subsequent digestion of carbohydrates farther along in the digestive tract. The slow release of carbohydrates caused by green tea prevents sharp peaks of blood insulin levels, which in turn favors fat burning over fat storage. Additionally, the extra levels of unabsorbed carbohydrates in the stool can benefit dieters by bulking the stools and helping to prevent constipation, a common complaint of dieters.

Although the body of literature is small for green tea as a diet aid, preliminary studies are promising. Reporting in the journal *Agricultural & Biological Chemistry,* scientists at the Food Research Laboratories of Mitsui Norin Co. in Shizuoka, Japan, indicated that polyphenols extracted from green tea inhibit the activity of amylase at much lower dosages than that found in just one cup of green tea. Further research is continuing in this area, particularly since it is "of great interest if tea polyphenols could control body weight without sacrificing the appetite."[14]

One of the ways in which tea supports weight loss efforts is by slightly boosting the body's rate of burning calories.[15] This modest 3 to 4 percent increase in energy expenditure doesn't make tea a miracle weight loss pill, but it does give dieters an extra boost that can get them over a plateau or keep them motivated.

When French researchers provided green tea extract supplements to a group of moderately obese individuals for three months, their body weight dropped by 4.6 percent and their waist circumference went down by an average of almost 5 percent.[16] These numbers might sound small, but become impressive if you consider that other diet and exercise changes were not made.

When a group of men took green tea extract (containing 90 milligrams of EGCG three times a day), they burned 266 more calories every day than men taking placebos. Again, this small amount could really add up over time.[17]

When laboratory mice are fed either a low-fat or high-fat diet, the mice that also get supplemented with green tea extract don't gain as much weight on the high-fat diet when they are in the green tea extract group.[18]

Sixty obese middle-aged women were placed on a diet of 1,800 calories per day. Some of the women took green tea supplements with breakfast, lunch, and dinner; the others took placebo pills. After two weeks on this regimen, the women taking green tea extract had lost twice as much weight as the placebo group. Results were even more impressive after the full month of the trial; the green tea users had three times the weight loss of the women who were simply dieting.[19]

The caffeine content of green tea is part—but not all—of the reason that green tea promotes weight loss. Caffeine increases the body's basal metabolic rate (the rate at which energy is used for the basic functions of breathing, pumping blood, and maintaining body temperature). This increase is referred to as a thermogenic effect; it may boost weight loss by helping the body burn more calories during day-to-day life. The potential effect on weight loss is small, but significant.[20]

The Coca-Cola company has come out with a green tea product called Enviga. This is a ready-to-drink beverage that contains both EGCG and caffeine, as well as other plant extracts. It is touted to speed up metabolism and promote weight loss. But you can get the same effect, for just three cents a cup, by making yourself a cup of green tea at home.

Aside from being a tasty part of many meals, green tea is a healthful addition to the diet. Green tea acts as a digestive aid, is a source of important nutrients, such as vitamin C and fluoride, and protects the digestive tract from potentially harmful compounds found in some foods. In addition, green tea promotes the friendly bacteria needed for a healthy intestine, helps treat inflammatory bowel disease, and may even help prevent ulcers and aid weight-loss efforts. All in all, green tea is a great way to start—or end—almost any meal. The next chapter will show even more ways that green tea promotes good health for women.

chapter nine

Women, Brew Up
a Cup of Tea . . .

A s we've seen, the first clues to the health benefits of green tea for men came from the discovery that Japanese men enjoyed surprisingly low rates of incidence for many diseases. In a similar way, the low rates of breast cancer and osteoporosis in Japanese women suggested that green tea should be in every woman's teacup. As we'll see in this chapter, green tea can be a healthful addition for women throughout their life span. (See pages 154–55, however, for a caution about caffeine.)

. . . For Strong Bones

Throughout most of the stages of its development, osteoporosis is an invisible disease. It progresses without any obvious symptoms until irreversible pain, loss of height, change in posture, and bone fractures make it all too obvious. Osteoporosis develops when bones become overly porous and brittle from the loss of calcium and other minerals. More than 44 million Americans, four-fifths of them women, currently suffer from osteoporosis or have dangerously low bone mass. After age sixty-five, one-half of all women and one-fifth of all men break bones because of osteoporosis—accounting for millions of fractures every year.

Treatments for osteoporosis are few and have a low success rate, but the disease may be preventable. Strong, dense bones are the best defense against osteoporosis; exercising and maintaining optimal intake of calcium and other essential minerals throughout life shows great success in developing osteoporosis-resistant bones. During childhood and adolescence, adequate calcium and vitamin D in the diet are crucial for the development of strong, dense bones. During the middle years, when calcium loss from bones exceeds calcium gain to bones, dietary calcium may slow the rate of bone loss.

Bones undergo a continual process of remodeling, in which old bone is removed and new bone is deposited. When bone resorption, the removal of old bone, occurs at a faster rate than the depositing of new bone, osteoporosis is likely. For every man who develops osteoporosis, eight women do. Their relatively small bones and the hormonal changes that accompany menopause put women at greater risk for developing the disease. During and after menopause, dietary calcium is essential to prevent the rapid bone loss associated with the advanced stages of osteoporosis, yet the average woman consumes only half the recommended intake for calcium, and amounts that low are associated with bone loss and the development of osteoporosis.

According to a study of bone resorption in animals, catechins can reduce excessive resorption that could lead to excessive loss of bone mass. Epidemiological studies of human populations support this theory. In recognition of findings such as these, tea drinking has been identified by the Mediterranean Osteoporosis Study as a protective factor against osteoporosis.[1]

Even though higher intakes of caffeine have been suggested as a risk factor for lower bone mineral density, research indicates that that drinking tea does not adversely affect bone mineral density. Bone mineral density is an indicator of strong, osteoporosis-resistant bones. In fact, a few preliminary studies even suggest that tea actually has a beneficial role in bone health. Several studies have now shown that women who are regular tea drinkers tend to have higher bone mineral density than non–tea drinkers, and this effect is even stronger in women who have been habitual tea drinkers for the longest amount of time.[2] It seems that the flavonoids in tea could influence bone mass and thus tea drinking might reduce the risk of osteoporosis.

Green tea may also give hope to sufferers of another bone disorder, *osteogenesis imperfecta*. *Osteogenesis imperfecta* is a rare inherited disease in which the bones are abnormally brittle and fragile. Fractures are the main symptom, and the most severe cases are fatal. The only trea currently available is to take measures to reduce the risk of fractures. Clearly, other treatment options are anxiously awaited. Dr. G. Cetta reported that catechin supplements improved the bone structure and normalized the cartilage function of two patients with *osteogenesis imperfecta*. In a similar study, four girls aged four to twelve who were afflicted with the disease were treated with catechins over a period of several months. Their bone fractures greatly decreased in frequency, and microscopic analysis of their bones showed that many of the previously abnormal bone parameters had been normalized. Although further research is warranted, these case studies are promising.[3]

... For Protection Against Breast Cancer

In the 1950s, one American woman in twenty was at risk for developing breast cancer. Today, one in eight is at risk, and about 40,970 women die annually. Why are so many women suffering from this deadly disease? Researchers looking to answer this question have identified many risk factors—from a family history of breast disease to never having had children. (See "Breast Cancer Risk Factors," below.)

Epidemiologists suggested a link between green tea and a lower risk of breast cancer after noticing that the risk of breast cancer in Japanese

Breast Cancer Risk Factors

The risk factors for breast cancer are:

- a family history of breast cancer
- onset of menstruation before age twelve
- beginning menopause at a late age
- giving birth to a first child after age thirty
- never giving birth
- being 40 percent above normal weight for one's age and height

women who moved to the United States and adopted an American diet quickly rose from the very low risk for women in Japan to the much higher risk of an average American woman. It seems to follow that American women could lower their chances of becoming breast cancer statistics by emulating women in Japan and including green tea in their diets.

Laboratory studies into the relationship between green tea and breast cancer indicate that green tea extracts, and EGCG in particular, inhibit the growth of breast cancer cells in mice. The tea extracts accomplish this by interacting with tumor promoters, hormones, and growth factors to "seal off" the cancer cells. EGCG also slows the growth of breast cancer cells that would otherwise tend to grow abnormally fast, thereby contributing to the spread of the cancer.[4]

A Caution About Caffeine

Women who suffer from fibrocystic breast disease or premenstrual syndrome (PMS) and women who are pregnant may want to be cautious with their intake of tea, since some evidence suggests that the caffeine in tea can actually worsen these conditions.

At some point in their lives, more than half of all women report suffering from symptoms of fibrocystic breast disease, a condition characterized by painful, lumpy breasts. Its underlying cause remains unknown. Women who experience fibrocystic breast disease may be at greater risk for breast cancer later in life. Green tea, per se, is not implicated in this condition, but the caffeine that it contains is. In the early 1980s, one study suggested that caffeine leads to an increased risk of developing fibrocystic breast disease. As many as 65 percent of the women in this study experienced a complete alleviation of their symptoms when they eliminated coffee, tea, chocolate, and other sources of caffeine from their diets. Subsequent research has not replicated or confirmed any connection between caffeine and fibrocystic breast disease; nonetheless, some women who continue to avoid caffeine report an improvement in their symptoms.[5]

Premenstrual syndrome (PMS) is also only indirectly linked to the consumption of tea, since caffeine again appears to be the culprit. More than 150 symptoms have been documented in women suffering from PMS, but most PMS sufferers report symptoms of pain, mood changes, weight gain, swelling, breast tenderness, and cravings that develop one to fourteen days before menstruation. Some experts recommend avoiding any sources of caffeine to reduce the symptoms of PMS.

Dr. Annette MacKay Rossignol of Oregon State University teamed up with Chinese researchers at the Shanghai Medical University to investigate whether green tea influenced PMS. They followed the diets, green tea drinking habits, and PMS symptoms of 188 young Chinese women. Tea was the only source of caffeine for these women. Those who drank tea more frequently were found to be more likely to suffer from PMS, particularly if they drank five cups of green tea or more daily.

Although further research is needed before a definitive judgment can be made, it is very likely that caffeine is responsible for any adverse effects that female tea drinkers experience, including symptoms of fibrocystic breast disease and PMS; the other components of green tea are probably not implicated. If a woman feels that her fibrocystic breast disease symptoms or PMS symptoms are aggravated by caffeine, there is no reason why she couldn't drink decaffeinated tea or take caffeine-free green tea polyphenol supplements. Furthermore, if fibrocystic breast disease does increase the risk of breast cancer, it may be to her advantage to increase her intake of the cancer-fighting polyphenols found in green tea.[6]

Pregnant women should steer clear of all sources of caffeine, and, if possible, even avoid caffeine a few weeks before conception.

When researchers at the Nagoya City University Medical School in Nagoya, Japan, tested the anti-cancer potential of naturally occurring antioxidants, they discovered that green tea polyphenols came out on top in terms of preventing breast cancer. Groups of rats were exposed to carcinogens that greatly increase the risk of breast cancer while being fed a regular diet, or a diet augmented with one of several antioxidants. All of the antioxidants improved the survival rates of these animals through the thirty-six weeks of the study. Of the rats that developed breast cancer tumors, the rats in the green tea group had fewer and smaller tumors. The researchers concluded that "of the four antioxidants tested, the effects of GTC [green tea catechins] appeared most beneficial since no animals died of mammary tumor during the experiment. One interpretation is that GTC inhibited the growth of the mammary tumors."[7]

Australian researchers compared the diets of 1,009 women with breast cancer with those of 1,009 women without the disease: Regularly drinking tea reduced the risk of developing breast cancer.[8] And the longer time one has drunk tea, as well as the more cups consumed each day, correlated with greater protection. In short, the epidemiological data indicates the promising news that drinking five or more cups of green tea each day seems to correlate with breast cancer prevention.[9]

. . . For Protection Against Ovarian Cancer

Ovarian cancer is cancer that begins in the ovaries. This form of cancer has a relatively high mortality rate, in part because there are no early symptoms or easy screenings in place for it yet. Thus, it is often diagnosed at a much later stage. Although green tea is not a cure, it can play a role in preventing ovarian cancer. In a case-control study from China, the diets of 254 women with ovarian cancer were compared to that of 652 control women.[10] It was found that the risk for ovarian cancer decreased with the more frequently women drank tea, as well as the longer time period they had been habitual tea drinkers. Another study, this one in Sweden, recorded a detailed diet questionnaire from more than 61,000 women, age forty-plus.[11] After their health was tracked for more than fifteen years, cases of ovarian cancer were noted. It was clear that there was an inverse relationship between drinking tea and having ovarian cancer. In fact, for each additional cup of tea drunk daily, there was an 18 percent lower risk of developing ovarian cancer. Green tea, and EGCG in particular, appears to inhibit ovarian cancer growth by inducing cell death of cancerous cells (a process called apoptosis).[12]

When the 254 women from the Chinese study previously mentioned were followed during the three years following diagnosis, researchers noticed that how much tea they drank after diagnosis also had an effect.[13] For tea drinkers, almost 78 percent survived the three years after diagnosis, while only 48 percent of the non–tea drinkers were still alive after three years. It seems that it is not too late to benefit from green tea, even after diagnosis. Of additional interest during the treatment period, a different study found that adding EGCG to cancer cells in the laboratory increased the toxicity of the cancer drug cisplatin.[14]

In addition, the component unique to green tea, L-theanine, has been found to have benefits connected to ovarian cancer. Animal-based studies indicate that L-theanine shrinks the size of ovarian tumors (when given along with cancer-treating drugs), and lessens the chances of metastases to the liver. Finally, L-theanine was found to protect healthy, non-cancerous cells from the damaging effects of chemotherapy drugs.[15]

. . . For Healthy Skin

Healthy skin is an important aspect of beauty, but sun, gravity, free-radical damage, and a poor diet take their toll on healthy, youthful-looking skin. Because skin cells have a very short life span, only a few days, the skin is one of the earliest indicators of changes in nutrition. On the one hand, nutrient deficiencies soon produce skin problems; on the other hand, proper nutrition can have a quick and powerful effect on correcting problems.

Collagen, the skin's structural protein, gives young skin its firm, youthful appearance. The interlacing of collagen with elastin (a protein found in the body's elastic tissues) gives skin its strength, elasticity, and smoothness. When free radicals attack collagen, they damage the molecules that determine the skin's appearance and so contribute to an older-looking face. In addition, the enzyme collagenase breaks down collagen. The energy in the sun's ultraviolet rays can turn susceptible stable molecules into free radicals and therefore are a major threat to firm, youthful skin. Frequent or prolonged sun exposure is a major contributor to premature aging and wrinkles.

Green tea in general and EGCG by itself have both been studied for their impressive skin protection, particularly in the areas of averting photoaging of the skin and thwarting cancer-promoting changes to the skin caused by UV light.[16]

Psoriasis, a chronic inflammatory skin condition, causes itching and discomfort during flare-ups; 150,000 new cases are diagnosed every year. One treatment for moderate to severe cases of psoriasis is phototherapy (exposure to ultraviolet A radiation) while taking a medication called psoralens, which increases the skin's sensitivity to the light. This treatment, although highly effective, unfortunately can increase the chances of skin cancer. Research indicates that applying green tea extract both before and after the treatment can help minimize DNA damage to the skin that would otherwise contribute to the risk of cancer.[17]

Antioxidants, including the flavonoids, protect the skin from free radical damage. Flavonoids in general are well known for supporting healthy collagen and elastin and maintaining their elasticity. In part, they do this by realigning these proteins to a more youthful, undamaged form. Among the polyphenols in green tea, EGCG and ECG show the strongest effect in reducing collagenase activity. Supplementing the diet with antioxidants, such as green tea's polyphenols, lessens the likelihood of wrinkles.[18]

Allergies that produce skin reactions are a common affliction, affecting 15 percent of the population. Symptoms can manifest in many parts of the body; skin irritations, rashes, and swelling are common indications of allergic reactions. Green tea can help alleviate such allergy symptoms in several ways: by reducing inflammation, inhibiting the release of histamine from cells, and lessening the release of other allergy-mediated chemicals in the body.[19]

Some women may recall hosting "tea parties" as young girls. The research indicates that continuing this tradition—with green tea—might be a good idea for supporting the health and beauty of most adult women. Green tea is linked to maintaining strong bones, reducing the risk of breast and ovarian cancers, and sustaining young-looking skin. However, pregnant women and women whose premenstrual syndrome or fibrocystic breast disease worsens after caffeine ingestion will want to choose decaffeinated varieties of green tea or caffeine-free green tea supplements.

chapter ten

A Cup a Day Keeps the Dentist Away

Few parts of the body play such a variety of roles in everyday living as your mouth and teeth do. They are important for expressing yourself through speaking, singing, and smiling, but in a function even more basic to sustaining health, the teeth and mouth are responsible for the first phase of digesting food. The teeth break food into smaller pieces, and digestive enzymes mix with food in the mouth. The leading cause of tooth loss in people of all ages is tooth decay. By making the mouth inhospitable to the bacteria that cause tooth decay and by supporting healthy tooth enamel, green tea can make a valuable contribution to a plan for maintaining good dental health.

The Teeth

Although we may seem to be born toothless, the development of our teeth is well underway by the third month of pregnancy. After birth, the teeth do not begin to erupt through the gums until about six or seven months of age. Most children have a full set of twenty teeth by the age of three. The process of shedding these primary teeth and replacing them begins at about the age of five or six and continues through the elementary school years until there are twenty-eight adult, permanent teeth. An additional four teeth, the wisdom teeth, emerge in early adulthood to bring the total to thirty-two.

There are several kinds of teeth (incisors, canines, premolars, and molars), but each has the same basic structure. The part of the tooth that is visible above the gum line is the crown; it is covered with a layer of hard enamel to protect the tooth. Despite its indestructible appearance, enamel cannot heal itself once it has been injured or has become decayed. The next layer of the tooth under the enamel, dentin, is also a hard material, but not as hard as enamel. Unlike enamel, dentin is sensitive to hot and cold temperatures and to touch. If a tooth feels sensitive or painful, some area of enamel has been disturbed, exposing the dentin. Below the gum level, dentin is covered by a layer called cementum, and connective tissue connects the cementum to the jaw bone. At the center of the tooth is a cavity containing dental pulp, which includes blood vessels, nerves, lymph vessels, and connective tissue.

The Causes of Dental Cavities

First, the good news: Americans are taking better care of their teeth than ever before. Tooth decay has decreased in children over the years, and the number of children with cavities is dropping every year. The bad news? Almost every person will develop some dental caries (that is, tooth decay), usually before adulthood.

Some types of bacteria are always in the mouth; they are nurtured by food fragments that adhere to teeth. Tooth decay is initiated by the demineralization of the outer surface of the tooth as a result of acids produced by bacteria that digest carbohydrates. Decay of the tooth progresses as the tooth continues to lose minerals and the bacterial metabolites continue to act on the tooth. A cavity forms, which, if untreated, can grow and destroy the entire tooth and even the surrounding gum tissues.

Although there are more than eighty kinds of bacteria living in the average mouth, the species that is the number-one culprit in dental caries is *Streptococcus mutans,* called *S. mutans* for short. This microorganism is present in the majority of mouths around the globe. *S. mutans*'s favorite habitat is the surfaces of teeth, particularly the hard-to-reach spaces between adjoining teeth, although it is also commonly found on the chewing surfaces of teeth.

S. mutans converts sugar and other carbohydrates into acids, which become part of the sticky deposit called dental plaque. Plaque consists of many bacteria living together in a paste of sugars, proteins, saliva, and decomposing food particles. Plaque adheres to the teeth, and is especially likely to build up next to the gum line, and within the gum space (between the tooth and the gum), and in the areas where teeth touch.

Dentists and microbiologists are increasingly aware of the phenomenon of biomass. In contrast to free-living bacteria (called planktonic bacteria) that live as individual cells, some bacteria, especially those involved in dental plaque, form large colonies that cling together in a mat that includes a number of protein and carbohydrate components. Bacteria living in such biomasses are frequently insensitive to the antibiotics that readily kill planktonic bacteria since the biomass is very hard for most antibiotics to penetrate.

The acids in the plaque attack the minerals in the tooth's outermost surface, leading to erosion and the formation of tiny cavities in the enamel. These early cavities are unnoticeable, but they create a microenvironment that is particularly hospitable to the bacteria and their foodstuffs and is progressively harder to clean. As time goes on and the plaque continues to eat away at the tooth's enamel, you may feel pain when you eat something that is sweet, very cold, or very hot. At this point, the cavity has progressed considerably. When the bacteria reach the dentin, it may become inflamed; the inflammation puts pressure on the sensitive pulp, and you experience the pressure as a toothache.

Tooth decay is a slow but steady process. From the first tiny cavity to the onset of toothache, a cavity generally takes a year or two to develop in permanent teeth, slightly less time in children's teeth. The formation of a cavity can begin just twenty minutes after eating, the time it takes for bacteria to form acids from the food you eat. Short of not eating, there isn't much you can do about this stage of cavity development. However, the mouth is not without its defenses. Your saliva and the actions of your tongue wash away many of the leftover food particles before bacteria can utilize them for destructive purposes. Tooth brushing and flossing help remove the plaque where bacteria thrive, especially in the tight spaces between the teeth and at the gum line.

Tooth decay most often occurs on the chewing surfaces of the back teeth, since the chewing surfaces of molars, which are rougher than the surfaces of other teeth, provide places for food particles and bacteria to accumulate. Another common location for cavities to develop is between the teeth, since it is difficult to reach this area with a toothbrush and remove plaque. In adults, an increasing problem is "root caries," decay that develops at the base of a tooth, often precipitated by a receding gum line. Cavities are also prone to develop under an old filling or along the edge of a new filling if the edges were not sealed adequately.

The Dangers of a Sweet Tooth

People and plaque-promoting bacteria have something in common: They both love sweets. Though the bacteria in your mouth thrive on all types of sugar, they seem to grow best on a diet of sucrose, ordinary white table sugar. The prevalence and severity of dental cavities took a sharp upward swing in the middle of the nineteenth century, corresponding to a rapid rise in the consumption of sugar. Moreover, a higher rate of cavities appears suddenly in countries that change from diets traditionally low in sugar to a Western diet high in sugar. In a comparison of ninety countries, the amount of sugar in the diet was found to account for 28 percent of the causes of dental cavities.[1]

Pure sugar is not the only food that fuels the growth of dental plaque. Any digestible carbohydrate will do just fine as far as the bacteria are concerned, since they will progressively convert it to sucrose; this includes refined flour products and all sources of sugar, such as candy, honey, dried fruits, sweetened cereals, ice cream, canned or frozen fruits in syrup, hard candy, puddings, sodas, and other sweets. Since carbohydrates are an important part of our diet, they cannot be eliminated, but we can minimize their adverse dental effects and thereby discourage dental decay. New research indicates that the most important variable is not how much sugar is eaten, but how and when it is eaten. Specifically, sweet treats between meals do more harm than those eaten with a meal because the sugars are not diluted by other foods.

The following guidelines can minimize the tooth damage initiated by sugar:

- Choose your snacks carefully. Avoid chewy, sticky foods, especially as between-meal snacks. Bacteria love sweet and sticky foods. Candy, raisins, and dried fruit can cling to the teeth. This doesn't mean that you can never eat these foods, but you should brush your teeth after eating them.

- Time your snacks carefully. Nibbling throughout the day gives bacteria a constant food supply.
- Brush your teeth within twenty minutes after eating (because acid production by bacteria reaches its peak in this time). If you can't brush, at least rinse your mouth with water or green tea after a snack.

The Value of Fluoride Protection

Many years ago, dental researchers noticed that people living in areas of the country where fluoride occurred naturally in the drinking water had almost no cavities. Today it is a recognized fact that tooth decay is less prevalent in areas where fluoride occurs naturally or is added to the drinking water. The fluoridation of municipal water supplies, which began in the 1950s, now covers more than half of the United States population. Experts recommend one part per million of fluoride in water as a health-enhancing level. When fluoride levels are too high, harmless but unattractive brown stains can appear on the teeth. Levels of fluoride in excess of eight parts per million can result in the discoloration of teeth and, possibly, in bone abnormalities.

At appropriate levels, fluoride is good for teeth and contributes to bone structures that are harder, larger, more uniform, and more resistant to decay by acids and demineralization. The benefits of fluoride are greatest when exposure to it begins in infancy and continues during the development of a child's teeth. As many as half of all cavities could be prevented with optimal fluoride exposure. Many people, whether their water is fluoridated or not, have their dentists apply fluoride topically and use toothpastes with fluoride, which also provide some dental benefits.[2]

Green tea is an abundant source of fluoride, which partially accounts for its cavity-fighting properties. Tea plants accumulate fluoride from the soil into tea leaves as they grow, so the oldest tea leaves contain the highest levels of fluoride. As such, green and white teas (which are made from young leaves) do not contain as much fluoride as some other teas. Keep in mind that the water used to brew tea also contributes fluoride to the final cup. So the natural fluoride levels of your area will, in part, affect the final fluoride level of your cup of tea.

Scientists at the Dayalbagh Educational Institute in Agra, India, assessed the amount of fluoride provided by several types of tea. They found that powdered tea leaches more fluoride into a cup of tea than whole-leaf tea does. Brewing time also affects fluoride levels; maximum levels are reached after six minutes of steeping. In all, the scientists at Dayalbagh determined that a cup of tea contributes 0.3 to 1.9 milligrams of fluoride to the diet.[3] The recommended intake of fluoride for adults is 1.5 to 4.0 milligrams daily, so drinking green tea in moderation can go a long way toward meeting this goal.

Interestingly, researchers recently ran some experiments to further pinpoint the fluoride levels in tea.[4] When they brewed tea (regular tea purchased from a store) in low-fluoride water, fluoride from the tea leaves was readily released into the cup of tea. But when high-fluoride water was used, the tea leaves, instead of releasing any fluoride, actually absorbed fluoride from the water. It seems that with tea, you'll always get the right amount of fluoride. All in all, it appears that fortuitously, the amount of fluoride in an average cup of tea is on par with the amount recommended for U.S. water supplies for the goal of preventing cavities.[5]

Green tea provides fluoride protection in two ways. First, the process of drinking the tea exposes the surfaces of the teeth to fluoride in a process similar to rinsing the mouth with anti-plaque mouthwash or toothpaste. Second, after the green tea is swallowed the fluoride can be incorporated into the tooth structure.

The Effect of Green Tea on Cavities

In China and Japan, it is customary to take some green tea after every meal, a habit that is believed to maintain a healthy mouth. The merits of this traditional method of preventive medicine are being demonstrated by modern research that reveals the many ways in which green tea is friendly to the teeth. First and foremost, green tea inhibits the growth of S. mutans and other bacteria associated with plaque.[6] Chinese dental researchers reported in the Chinese Journal of Stomatology (stomatology is the study of dental health) that S. mutans growth was completely inhibited after just five minutes of contact with sufficient concentrations of polyphenols from green tea. Similar lines of research have demonstrated that green tea extracts prevent the cellular growth of S. mutans in laboratory dishes.[7] Other test tube studies confirm that green tea extract, as well as black and oolong tea extracts, are all able to inhibit the growth of cavity-producing bacteria.[8]

Researchers from the Department of Clinical Pathology at the Nihon University School of Dentistry in Japan investigated the cavity-preventing ability of green tea extracts in laboratory experiments and in studies of animals. In the laboratory, they grew S. mutans bacteria on saliva-coated discs that simulated teeth. They determined that polyphenols from green tea prevented the bacteria from attaching themselves to the simulated teeth and interfered with enzymes used by the bacteria to feed on sugar. EGCG was the most powerful cavity fighter of the polyphenols. When the researchers infected rats with S. mutans and fed them a diet known to contribute to dental cavities, they found that the rats were much less likely to develop cavities when they were also given polyphenol supplements.[9] Researchers at the New York University Dental Center tested the role of black tea extract on the development of dental cavities in an animal model. Hamsters who had their water fortified with black tea extract experienced 63.7 percent fewer cavities.[10]

Enzymes produced by S. mutans for the purpose of utilizing dietary sugars are highly related to the cavity-causing ability of this bacterium. These enzymes allow the bacteria to form larger areas of plaque on the tooth surface, which in turn lead to the formation of cavities. Polyphenols extracted from tea can lessen the risk of cavities by arresting the production of one of these enzymes, called glucosyltransferase. When polyphenols are added to their drinking water, animals develop far fewer cavities and accumulate less plaque. Researchers from the Department of Oral Microbiology at Osaka University in Japan say that fewer cavities develop because the polyphenols block production of glucosyltransferase by the bacteria.[11]

Another investigation conducted by the same research group examined the effects of tea polyphenols on plaque deposition in human subjects. At the start of this study, thirty-five volunteers aged eighteen to twenty-nine were given thorough dental examinations and the level of bacteria in their mouths was measured. Then, for each of two four-day periods, the volunteers followed experimental oral hygiene procedures. In the first period, they ate a normal diet but refrained from all oral hygiene other than rinsing their mouths with a solution containing tea polyphenols after each meal and before bed. In the second period, they followed the same regimen, but the mouth rinse did not contain any active ingredients. At the end of each study period, bacteria counts were taken again and another dental examination was conducted. In thirty-four of the thirty-five volunteers, plaque deposition was clearly decreased by rinsing with the tea polyphenols, even though the volunteers were not brushing or flossing, suggesting that polyphenols have powerful anti-plaque properties. No adverse side effects were reported by the study participants.[12] In other research, a cross-section study of more than 6,000 British school children (fourteen years old) determined that the teens who drank tea experienced fewer cavities than non–tea drinkers. This benefit of tea was not affected by whether or not sugar was added to the tea.[13]

Green tea polyphenols also reduce the risk of cavities by increasing the resistance of the tooth to the actions of cavity-causing bacteria. Researchers at the Department of Preventive Dentistry, Kyushu University, Japan, have concluded that green tea given along with fluoride results in an enamel tooth surface that is more highly resistant to acids produced by bacteria than the tooth surface that results when fluoride alone is used.[14]

Statistical comparisons show that the dental health of children who drink at least one cup of tea daily is better than that of children who drink less than three cups per week. Other research in school-age children indicates that drinking green tea reduces the number of cavities.[15]

In all of the studies that compare the cavity prevention of the various polyphenols, EGCG consistently emerges as the most powerful protector of dental health of all the polyphenols. A cup of green tea generally contains 50 to 100 milligrams of polyphenols; since this is a greater dose of polyphenols than that used in the studies discussed in this section, regular consumption of moderate amounts of green tea has great potential for stopping dental cavities in their tracks and keeping teeth as healthy as possible.

Even if preventive measures have failed and a cavity has developed, green tea can still help. According to traditional healers, the pain of a toothache can sometimes be eased by gently chewing tea leaves or simply pressing the tea leaves against the tooth in question. Meanwhile, of course, you'll want to contact your dentist.

If the root canal has become infected, green tea may help prevent further damage. Polyphenol extracts from four different Japanese green teas (ordinary, refined, coarse, and roasted) were assessed for their antibacterial effects against twenty-four different strains of bacteria found in infected root canals. The researchers hypothesized: "If Japanese green teas could be shown to have an antibacterial effect on various bacteria detected in infected root canals, then they may be a possible medicament

The Ideal Plaque Fighter

In an article in the *Dental Clinics of North America,* Dr. Michael Bral of the New York University College of Dentistry outlined nine qualities of an ideal anti-plaque agent.[16] They were:

- eliminates disease-causing bacteria only
- does not lead to the development of resistant bacteria
- stays in the mouth for an extended period of time
- is safe
- reduces plaque and gingivitis
- does not stain teeth
- has no adverse effects on teeth
- is easy to use
- is inexpensive

Dr. Bral noted that no agent met all of these criteria. In fact, most potential agents fail in several areas. While green tea is not perfect, it meets eight of these nine criteria for an ideal anti-plaque agent, which is impressive (it doesn't ordinarily stay in the mouth for an extended period of time). Overall, green tea's beneficial dental qualities add up to a great opportunity for preventive dental care.

for use in the treatment of the infected canals." True to form, the poly-phenols came through as antibacterial agents in this study. The green teas inhibited the growth of as many as half of the bacteria strains, sug-gesting that green tea may indeed be a promising adjunct in treatment for infected root canals.[17]

The Effect of Green Tea on Gum Disease

Gingivitis is the inflammation of the gingiva, that is, the gums. Its symp-toms are swollen, soft, red gums that bleed easily. This condition often goes unnoticed since it is usually painless. In most cases, gingivitis results from poor dental hygiene practices; proper daily brushing and flossing and regular dental cleanings greatly decrease the chances of developing gingivitis. When gingivitis progresses untreated, periodontal disease can develop.

In periodontal disease, plaque-filled pockets form between the teeth and gums. The gums become inflamed, enlarging these pockets and trapping even more plaque. Over time, the gums detach from the teeth, pus forms as a result of the infection, and the affected tooth loosens and may even fall out.

Gingivitis is reversible, but the damage done by periodontal disease is permanent; that is why treatment for gingivitis is absolutely crucial for continuing dental health. Gingivitis is often caused by the same bacterial plaque that causes dental cavities, so green tea's effectiveness against that bacteria not only prevents cavities but can also result in a reduced risk for gingivitis. Other bacteria, specific to gingivitis, are also inhibited by green tea. Like conventional treatments for gum disease, green tea is most effective at the earliest stage of development, and is probably ineffective if gingivitis progresses to the serious condition of periodontal disease.

The Effect of Green Tea on Bad Breath

Plaque not only causes tooth decay and gum disease but is also the pri-mary cause of bad breath. The odor of bad breath, or halitosis as it is technically called, comes from a combination of bacteria, decomposing food, and decomposing tissue. Although bad breath has been blamed on many foods, such as garlic, onions, and cheese, no food does more than temporarily increase preexisting bad breath caused by plaque. If plaque is removed daily through brushing and flossing, and decayed teeth are cleaned and repaired, most cases of bad breath will be alleviated. Rinsing the mouth with green tea, or even simply swishing a mouthful of green tea around your mouth, can aid in the prevention and treatment of bad breath by dislodging accumulated bacteria and food particles and decreasing the amount of plaque on the teeth.

If your mouth and teeth are pain-free, that's great, but the absence of pain does not mean that your mouth and teeth are completely healthy. The development of any disease progresses along a continuum from health to severe illness. The early stages of dental disease are undetectable, but they are the first missteps on a path that leads to tooth decay and gum disease. Good oral hygiene (brushing twice a day and flossing daily) and twice-yearly visits to a dentist for preventive care are crucial elements of a good dental plan. Adding green tea is a painless and tasty way to help keep the mouth and teeth healthy.

chapter eleven

It's Tea Time!

It's refreshing, stimulating, and health-enhancing; that's why tea is the most popular beverage in the world (after water). Overall tea consumption, worldwide, averages four fluid ounces per person every day, though pockets of tea enthusiasts, such as the Japanese, Chinese, and British, account for disproportionately large tea intakes. Tea is safe to consume over a wide range of levels of intake; in fact, populations with typically higher levels of tea consumption are consistently shown to have derived greater health benefits from the tea they drink. To make drinking tea even easier, there are many varieties of tea, so there's sure to be a tea to please almost any palate.

Finding the Right Amount

How much green tea (or green tea extract) you should consume to benefit your health depends on your overall diet, your lifestyle, and the presence or absence of risk factors, such as smoking or a family history of heart disease. To achieve the health benefits noted in Asian countries, it would seem that a person should consume at least as much as people there do. The average green tea intake in Asian countries is about three cups daily, which means an intake of 240 to 320 milligrams of polyphenols. In short, the "right" number for tea seems to be about three to six cups daily. Research shows that this amount will lower your risk of everything from heart attack, skin cancer, and breast cancer to stroke. But keep in mind that there is not a threshold effect; that is, drinking less than three cups will not be without merit. Any amount of tea you drink will convey health benefits.

Scientific studies of green tea generally indicate that the dose of polyphenols needed for effective health protection is 300 to 400 milligrams of polyphenols or more daily, usually taken in the form of a green tea extract that may be standardized up to 97 percent polyphenols (with up to 67 percent being EGCG). Lesser dosages are required for green tea extracts with higher EGCG contents. These dosages are equivalent to four to ten cups of green tea daily.

The long history of human consumption of tea, particularly green tea, with apparent safety confirms that tea is safe to use in reasonable doses. In fact, the Food and Drug Administration (FDA) has certified it as safe, listing it on the Generally Recognized As Safe (GRAS) list and accepting it as a flavoring agent. The safety of green tea extract is impressive; even several hundred times more than a normal amount of green tea does not produce adverse reactions. The most common adverse effect from exceptionally high tea consumption is overstimulation brought on by caffeine, leading to such disturbances as insomnia. Anyone sensitive to this effect should restrict intake of caffeine from all sources. Fortunately, decaffeinated tea products are available, as are caffeine-free dietary supplements.

Can you drink too much tea? Well, it is hard to do, but it is possible. For example, when an elderly woman drank the equivalent of almost twenty-nine 3.5-ounce cups of oolong tea daily, she developed abnormally low potassium levels.[1] This problem was thought to be a result of the tea's caffeine levels. Another theoretical problem related to very high tea intakes (again this would be excessive amounts that very few people would be inclined to drink) is a potential interaction with the blood thinning drug warfarin (Coumadin). One case report of this happening involved a person who drank up to a gallon of green tea daily. At this enormous level of intake, the small amount of vitamin K in green tea can add up, which is the probable source of interaction with the blood-thinning drug. The average person's intake of green tea is not thought to be a problem, even for those taking warfarin.[2]

Making the Supplement Choice

The unique aroma and taste of green tea are appreciated around the world, but some people simply don't care for it as a beverage or don't want to drink the quantity of tea every day that is associated with disease prevention and treatment. For anyone who does not want to drink green tea every day—for reasons of convenience, taste, caffeine content, or any other reason—green tea extracts in supplement form are a great alternative. In addition to EGCG supplements, there are also L-theanine supplements available in the marketplace.

Throughout this book we have shown that the polyphenols from green tea offer a multitude of health benefits. We think there is every reason to become a tea drinker, but if green tea isn't "your cup of tea," green tea extracts are available that offer the benefits of green tea in the convenience of a capsule. Supplemental forms of green tea extract provide polyphenols in a controlled dosage form, so you know exactly how much you're getting. On the other hand, when you brew a cup of tea, the polyphenol levels can vary as a result of many factors, including where the tea plant was grown, how it was processed, its age, and how you brewed it. When choosing a green tea extract supplement, look for one that is decaffeinated and has a high polyphenol content.

Tea Shopping Guide

It used to be that having a cup of tea meant a quick dunk of a stale tea bag into a teacup. No longer. The world of tea has expanded to include "real" teas that come in black, green, oolong, or white varieties, as well as tisanes, or infusions, of any number of herbs that are chosen for their intriguing flavors and myriad of health benefits (see "What's in Your Cup?" on page 8). Of course, the herbal tisanes do not provide the same benefits as true teas, but they can be a tasty alternative every once in a while.

It's easier than it's ever been to find high-quality teas. In fact, there are more than 2,000 specialty tea salons and retail shops across the United States, in both big cities and small towns, and this number will just be increasing in the coming years. Today, gourmet teas are increasingly found in coffee houses, restaurants, health food stores, mainstream supermarkets, drug stores, and—just as they've always been—Asian markets.

It should come as no surprise if you feel daunted by the number of choices when selecting a tea. To a certain extent, you can simply let your tastes guide you, since all teas are going to provide health benefits. Thus, there's nothing wrong with grabbing a container of generic green tea and brewing up a cup. However, if you want to dip your toe deeper in the water and become more of a tea connoisseur, the myriad of choices you have available can come as quite a shock (there can be hundreds!) the first time you enter a tea salon. To make that job a little easier you can ask yourself these six questions, which will help you narrow down the choices and determine the price you'll pay:

Question	Effect on price
1. How important is tea quality?	Higher tea grades more expensive
2. Do you prefer loose-leaf tea or tea bags?	Tea bags more expensive than loose
3. Do you want caffeinated or decaffeinated?	Generally no price difference
4. Do you care if it's organic or Fair Trade?	Organic/Fair Trade more expensive
5. Which tea varieties taste better to you?	Price varies greatly by tea variety
6. Are you interested in herb-blended teas?	Generally no price difference

And now, a closer look at these questions:

1. Do you care about tea quality?

Teas are graded according to their quality. Finer quality teas are the most expensive and are distinguished by the presence of tea leaf tips in the finished product. In general, whole leaves are graded more highly, and as the leaf fragments are broken more and more, the grade declines. In descending order, the major tea grades are:

Broken Orange
Pekoe
Broken Pekoe Souchong
Broken Orange Pekoe
Fannings
Dust

2. Do you prefer loose-leaf tea or tea bags?

Traditionally, tea is brewed from loose leaves and there is an argument for loose tea conveying more antioxidants. Tea bags necessarily use the smaller bits of leaves (fannings and dust) that are considered lower quality, so that they can adequately infuse through the bag.

However, there can be no argument that tea bags offer convenience in both tea preparation and ease of disposal of spent leaves. Which is surely why tea bags became an instant hit when they were first introduced back in 1904, and today their popularity remains strong. On a per-serving basis, tea bags tend to be more expensive than loose leaves, since part of the price goes to packaging rather than quality tea. In addition, you should consider whether the packaging itself of the tea bag (and inks used in some tea bags) conveys a noticeable taste and unwanted addition to your cup of tea. For most people it comes down to a question of taste versus convenience. If you find a bagged tea that tastes good to you, then the convenience may be worth it.

3. Do you want caffeinated or decaffeinated?

If you choose decaffeinated tea for health reasons, you might be interested to know that there are several methods that can be used to remove the caffeine from tea leaves—and they are not all created equal.

There are two main methods in use. The first one uses a solvent such as ethyl acetate, while the other relies on carbon dioxide and water. It probably won't come as a surprise that we favor the carbon dioxide/water method, with one of the reasons being it only minimally affects EGCG levels, while the solvents can remove and/or destroy most of the EGCG in tea. Incidentally, the carbon dioxide used in this method is solid ("dry ice") under pressure, which means that after the treatment process it evaporates and does not leave any residue in the tea. The label of the tea should state which decaffeination method was used; if not you can contact the manufacturer to inquire as to their caffeine removal process.

4. Do you care if it's organic or Fair Trade?

Organic teas, like other organic foods and beverages in the marketplace, are grown and manufactured according to National Organic Standards established by the U.S. Department of Agriculture. Organic teas will be labeled as such, and certified by a USDA-approved independent agency (such as Quality Assurance International, Inc.), so you know that the tea was grown without pesticides or chemicals. Think of it as your green tea going really green. Organic teas do cost a bit more, but many consumers find the environmental and social benefits worth it.

Fair Trade certification relates specifically to work conditions of the tea workers. Fair Trade farmers are supported by getting a fair price for the tea product. They can then invest in the farming community to improve health care, education, and housing for their families. Fair Trade certification builds a partnership between the tea farmer, tea trader, and you—the tea drinker. The cycle becomes positive and sustainable for all involved. It likely costs a little more to buy a Fair Trade tea, but it should pay off in the future.

5. Which tea varieties taste better to you?

Here you're just going to have to follow your palate. All of the green teas confer substantial health benefits—the slight differences are not enough to drink a tea that doesn't suit your tastes. Cost of the tea reflects not just tea quality, but whether the tea variety is rare (or rarely exported). You may find that you like a moderately priced variety more than an expensive one so price will not always be an indicator of "better" teas. After tasting a few varieties of tea, you'll start to notice certain qualities you tend to like—fruity, rich, delicate, floral, and so on, and you can look for new teas that have those qualities. See "Green Tea Varieties" below for detailed descriptions of the main varieties of tea you're likely to find in tea salons and other markets selling tea.

Tea varieties are a bit like wine vintages. People with highly trained tongues can readily tell the taste difference between vintages and brands of the same kind of wine (merlots, for example) and develop preferences for which they are willing to pay premium prices. Others are less discriminating. So it is with tea. Find a brand or style that pleases you and do not be intimidated by those who have arrived at a different preference.

6. Are you interested in herb-blended teas?

There are many green teas available that are combined with any number of herbs. You'll still get the health benefits of the green tea, but the herbs add an interesting taste dimension to the brew. Green tea combined with mint is among the more commonly found herb blends. Other readily available herbs blended with green tea include echinacea, ginseng, and ginger.

Scented green teas are also plentiful. Jasmine green tea, for example, is made by allowing green tea to absorb the scent and flavor of jasmine flowers. Jasmine tea has a fragrant aroma and refreshing taste. Other scented teas include orchid, plum, gardenia, rose, mango, lavender, apricot, strawberry, and lychee. Rooibos (red bush tea) is another addition to some green tea products, resulting in a more fruity taste (as well as additional health benefits).

Green Tea Varieties

Sifting through the sea of green tea choices can be overwhelming. The following descriptions will let you know a bit about the main types that are available, organized by country of origin.

Chinese Green Teas

CHUN MEE: Green tea leaves are twisted into curved shapes, thus earning it the name "precious eyebrows." The tea leaves themselves have a dusty appearance and the taste is less sweet than many other green teas.

DRAGON PEARLS: This green tea has a sweet, nutty taste. The leaves are formed into balls that unfurl as they steep—a lovely sight to watch.

DRAGON WELL: This is one of China's favorite and most popular green teas. The name refers to a legendary well in the region of China producing this tea. Dragon Well tea has a lively green color, brisk taste, and somewhat earthy aroma. The tea leaves appear bright and shiny and are smooth to the touch. With the addition of hot water, the leaves open up to reveal intact buds within. Also called Lung Ching.

EMERALD PETALS: Tea made of delicate flat green leaves; no stems or buds are included in the final product. The brewed tea tastes smooth and has a floral aroma. It's grown in Lu An county of Anhui province and is also known as Lu An Gua Pian.

GREEN PEONY: This tea is hand-made by tea artisans who select large tea buds and tie them with silk thread to resemble a peony flower. When hot water is added (never use boiling water for this delicate tea), the "flower" will open. The brewed tea has a smooth, floral taste.

GUNPOWDER: When this type of green tea is processed, each leaf is rolled tightly into a pellet shape, which then unfurls when boiling water is poured over it. An employee of the British East India Company is reputed to have given this tea its name because he thought it resembled gunpowder (either because of its shape or its grayish-green color, or both). Since it is tightly rolled, Gunpowder green tea stays fresh for the longest storage time of the green teas. Be careful not to overbrew, or a bitter flavor can result. Properly brewed Gunpowder tea tastes fresh and grassy. Also called Pearl.

HYSON: This type of green tea was named for an East India merchant by the same name, who was the first to sell a certain type of green tea in England. The leaves used to make Hyson tea are thick and yellow-green; they are twisted into long, thin shapes during manufacture. It is one of the more pungent tasting green teas. Also called Young Hyson.

IMPERIAL: This is a rolled leaf tea made from older leaves. It is also grown and made in India and Sri Lanka.

JADE SPRING: A somewhat sweet-tasting green tea, it can be re-steeped without becoming bitter. The needle-shaped leaves of this tea variety have downy white hairs.

PI LO CHUN: This is a rare and famous green tea; the name translates as Green Snail Spring. The leaves are hand rolled and resemble tiny snails. Peach, apricot, and plum trees are planted among the tea bushes, and the tea leaves absorb the fruity scent before being plucked.

WHITE TEA: Similar to green tea, white tea is only lightly processed (as opposed to black teas) and retains very high antioxidant levels—in fact, slightly higher antioxidant levels compared to green teas. White teas are made from the youngest tea leaves and buds—silver-colored hairs can be seen on the tea buds. Brewed white tea has a very pale color and mild taste. White teas are primarily produced in the Fujian Province of China, and are more rare and costly than other teas. Also called Silver Tip or Silver Needles.

Japanese Green Teas

BANCHA: This tea is a lower quality form of Sencha. The leaves are more coarse and larger, generally because they are from the last plucking of the season. This tea is not generally exported from Japan. The brewed tea has a yellow-green color, and the flavor is full.

GENMAICHA: This Japanese specialty tea is made by blending green tea leaves with fire-roasted rice, so technically this tea is a blend. The resulting tea has a mild, slightly toasty, grainy taste. Sometimes called "popcorn" tea because a few grains of rice pop during the processing and can be seen in the final product.

GYOKURO: This tea has flat, sharply pointed leaves that resemble pine needles. The brewed tea is green, sweet, and smooth tasting. It has a reputation in Japan as being superior quality and its name means "precious dew." It's similar in appearance to Sencha, but a bit darker green with thicker leaves. The taste is smooth and less bitter than Sencha.

HOJICHA: This green tea is made from large, unrolled leaves that are pan fried or oven-roasted to produce an earthy aroma and nutty flavor. This process lessens bitter taste in the tea but unfortunately lowers the level of antioxidants as well. As such, it would not be the best choice for someone drinking green tea for health benefits.

MATCHA: Green tea leaves are pulverized into a powder for this tea. A beverage is made by whisking and dissolving the powder in hot water, rather than brewing the tea leaves themselves. The resulting beverage has a vibrant bright green color and light, sweet taste. Matcha is the tea used traditionally in the Japanese tea ceremony. Matcha can be added to desserts as well. Also called "froth of liquid jade."

SENCHA: Sencha is probably the most popular, easily found Japanese tea, and it is a good everyday drinking tea. Approximately 75 percent of Japan's tea production is of Sencha tea. The taste is slighty astringent, although there is an underlying sweetness as well. This tea has a light green color and fresh green scent.

Indian Green Tea

India primarily produces black teas, especially in the Assam region. However, small quantities of green and white tea are also grown here.

Korean Green Tea

Korean green teas are less readily available in Western countries, and thus the price tends to be higher. Korean green tea varieties include Ujeon, Sejak, and Jungjak.

Sri Lanka (Ceylon) Tea

The teas mostly grown in Sri Lanka are black teas. The names of most green teas grown in this area correspond with the names of Chinese green teas (such as Gunpowder). The green teas from this country tend to be a bit darker in color and richer in flavor.

Tibetan Green Tea

Tibet is probably best known for brick tea, which, as the name implies, is literally tea compressed into the shape of a brick. This process started as a better way for nomads to transport tea over long distances. Brick tea may be aged for many years and has an earthy mellowness and dark red color. Because of the long storage times, it is likely that the antioxidant levels in brick tea are lower than other green teas; again, for those with their eye on the health benefits of green tea, this is probably not the best everyday drinking choice. Also called pu-erh.

Vietnamese Green Tea

Black tea is a far more common export for Vietnam, but lots of green tea is grown (and drunk) in this country as well. One expensive specialty from Vietnam is lotus tea, made from green tea leaves placed inside a lotus flower for numerous hours. White tea is also produced here.

Black Teas

There are numerous black teas available in the marketplace. Although they contain lower levels of antioxidants compared to green tea, black teas certainly convey health benefits to those who prefer the taste. Common black teas include English Breakfast, Irish Breakfast, Ceylon Breakfast, Caravan, Darjeeling, Earl Grey, Assam, Keemun, Lapsang Soucho, and Pingsuey.

Still Unsure?

If you still don't know which tea to choose, you can't go wrong selecting a tea with a fresh, light color—since those are the teas most likely to have the highest antioxidant levels. You might also want to consider whether you'll be using the tea quickly or slowly (and choose hardier/ more delicate teas accordingly). And again, you should feel free to let your tastes dictate since all teas will provide some health benefits: It really is a no-lose proposition when you drink tea of any kind!

Remember that you can simply ask for a sample (or buy a small amount to try at home) before you commit to larger quantities of a tea that you may end up not liking. Even if you are partial to the most expensive tea, tea is a very affordable indulgence—since a pound of loose-leaf tea can make two-hundred cups.

Once Home . . .

Since the compounds contained in tea are air sensitive, try (as much as you can tell) to buy tea that has not been on the shelf for a long time. Good store practice involves placing newly arrived material at the back of the supply presented to the public so that materials do not stand a long time at the back of the line and become quite aged. This is not always followed, but the better stores do this.

The shelf life of tea varies based on storage conditions and variety. Black teas last longer than green teas, and certain specialty green teas (such as flower teas) are at their peak for as little as a month. (One exception is Pu-erh brick tea; its taste actually improves with age.) In general, black tea will keep for up to two years if stored in a dry, cool location in an airtight container, such as a sealed opaque canister. Aim to buy only the amount of green tea that you can use within six months to a year, after which green tea loses its freshness. Among the green teas, tightly rolled teas such as Gunpowder keep better than open-leafed varieties.

Any tea can last a bit longer with this trick: Place desiccant packets or oxygen-absorbing packets in with the tea or vacuum seal the container. Refrigerating or freezing is not recommended, however. You'll know your tea is starting to age if it seems less flavorful than when you first bought it, becomes moldy, or has a faint taste or odor from foods stored near the tea.

Brewing the Perfect Pot of Tea

Brewing a pot or cup of green tea is a simple process, but the most important things to keep in mind for green and white teas are these:

Use very hot but not boiling water (the teas are just too delicate) and steep for only for a few minutes (less than three minutes). Please note that these are general guidelines—if the tea you purchase has specific recommendations, it is probably best to follow those. (See "Brewing the Noble Leaf" on page 186.) Milk, sugar, lemon, and other flavorings are not generally added to green tea; it is simply enjoyed in its unaltered state.

The amount of caffeine in your cup of tea depends in part on how long you brew it. The shorter the brewing time, the less caffeine there will be in the tea you drink. For example, infusing tea leaves in hot water for three minutes results in a caffeine content of 20 to 40 milligrams, while just one minute more results in 40 to 100 milligrams of caffeine. The size of the leaves you use can also affect caffeine content. The tiny broken bits of tea leaves that fill a tea bag release twice as much caffeine as the equivalent amount of whole leaves.

Tea aficionados suggest that a separate teapot should be kept for the exclusive use of green tea, so the residual flavors of black or oolong tea do not cross over into the next batch, but most people do not notice any taste difference brewing all types of tea in the same teapot. It is important to clean the pot, when done, by rinsing with plain water only, rather than using cleansers that could affect the taste of later tea batches.

Water Quality

The taste of your final beverage can be greatly influenced by the quality of the water used in brewing. This is especially true in hard water areas where there are a significant amount of inorganic ions in the water or in areas subject to drought wherein the water becomes quite concentrated and has a definite flavor, which many people dislike.

Another potential problem is areas with heavily chlorinated water. This not only affects the taste of the tea but, because of the oxidant power of the chlorine, diminishes some of the antioxidant power of the tea. Distilled water tends to tastes flat, so you may want to avoid that kind of water as well.

The perfectionist may prefer to brew tea in non-carbonated mineral water in order to get a consistent taste. Mineral water has some added ions so that its taste is more appealing.

Tea and Milk: Yay or Nay?

In many parts of the world (with England leading the list), adding a dash of milk to a cup of black tea is common practice. Unfortunately, this practice might interfere with the antioxidant capabilities of tea. Some studies indicate that the proteins in milk bind with flavonoids, thus reducing their activity in the body. However, other research has not found an effect on antioxidant status in people drinking tea either with or without milk.

Since the current literature remains conflicted, it would be prudent for those who aim to maximize their antioxidant intake to avoid adding milk to their tea. If, however, someone is simply drinking tea as a pleasant beverage, then there's no harm in mixing in some milk—but realize that this practice might be diminishing the health benefits of tea.

Forms of Tea

Nowadays you don't even have to drink anything to get a dose of green tea goodness. Green tea is an increasingly common ingredient in skin care products, such as moisturizers, lotions, eye creams, and sunscreens; and there is even a new gum on the market (chewing one piece packs the antioxidant punch of two cups of green tea).

Putting Tea to Unusual Uses

Taking green tea internally is not the only way to benefit from this herb. Traditional healers in many Asian countries use green tea leaves externally to treat a variety of conditions. For instance, washing the face with leftover tea can be very cleansing for the skin, particularly for treating minor cases of acne and skin rashes. Green tea even has a mild disinfectant action for minor skin injuries. Feet afflicted with fungal infections can be bathed with strongly brewed tea over a period of several weeks. Then, to lessen the likelihood that the fungus infection will flare up again, dried tea leaves (used or fresh) are placed in the patient's socks when they are stored in a drawer. Washing the hair normally, and then rinsing it in strong tea leaves it shiny and soft. Fatigued eyes can be reinvigorated by a wash of very weak green tea.

There are even some new medical uses for green tea. Tissue banks collect and preserve tissues (such as skin for grafts, corneas, or heart valves) until they can be used in an ill person. The freezing temperatures that the tissues undergo can cause some injuries to the tissues. Researchers recently discovered that adding polyphenols from green tea to the tissues greatly lessens any injuries caused by the storage process.[3] In fact, the green tea–based solution even allows for tissues to be preserved for several months at room temperature. This has great potential for developing countries that may not have reliable systems for transporting and keeping tissues frozen.

Green tea can play interesting roles in cooking other than its usual role as a beverage. A unique effect can be achieved when tea is used in the preparation of hard-boiled eggs. First, boil the eggs in water; then crack the shells somewhat, add plenty of tea leaves to the water, and return the eggs to a boil. After they have cooled, peel the eggs and slice them to reveal unique coloring, fragrance, and flavor. You can also add tea leaves to the fuel used in the smoking of foods; they will impart a pleasant taste.

Leftover brewed tea can be put to use in many ways. If new wooden furniture has an unpleasant smell from the glue used to attach veneer, from lacquer, or from other chemicals, washing it in strong tea will lessen the odor. Used tea leaves can be tossed around the roots of flowering plants, particularly rose bushes, where they act as an excellent mulch. After they have been dried in the sun, accumulations of used tea leaves can be used to stuff pillows. In China, such pillows are reputed to result in an excellent night's sleep.

A smoldering tray of burning green tea leaves is reputed to drive away mosquitoes, but if the tea leaves fail in this regard, you can prepare a soothing salve for insect bites (and sunburn) by simply applying moist leaves to the afflicted area.

Brewing the Noble Leaf

Figure 1. Tea Ball

Back when tea was so costly that only royalty could afford it, tea was known as the "noble leaf." Today, fortunately, anyone can enjoy tea. To brew a single cup, all you need is a china or glass cup and a tea bag. If you favor loose tea, you can use a hinged and perforated stainless steel tea ball (shown in Figure 1). Simply open the ball, put in a spoonful of tea, drop the ball into a cup of freshly boiled water, pop a lid on the cup, and let the tea steep. You'll also find special tea mugs that are fitted with a perforated infuser and have their own lids (as shown in Figure 2).

Using a perforated stainless steel spoon (as shown in Figure 3) is the least satisfactory method of brewing a single cup of loose tea because the handle protrudes and there's no way to cover the cup so that the tea can steep properly. The best you can do with one of these spoons is stir, and that just won't give you a full-flavored cup of tea.

Figure 2. Tea Mug

Figure 3. Perforated Spoon

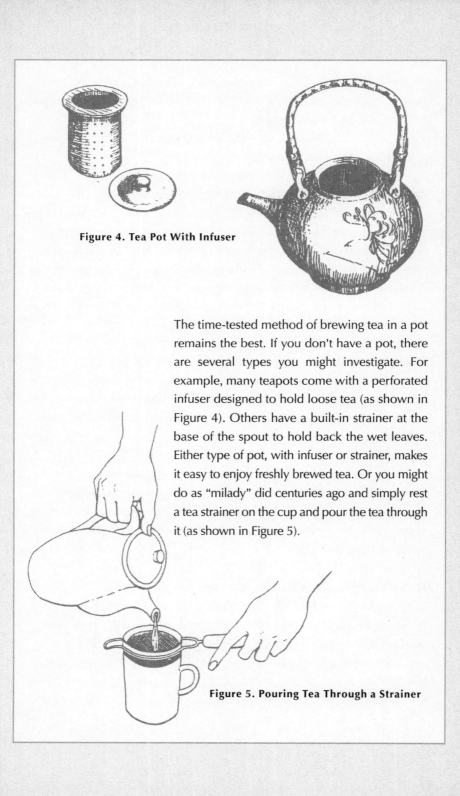

Figure 4. Tea Pot With Infuser

The time-tested method of brewing tea in a pot remains the best. If you don't have a pot, there are several types you might investigate. For example, many teapots come with a perforated infuser designed to hold loose tea (as shown in Figure 4). Others have a built-in strainer at the base of the spout to hold back the wet leaves. Either type of pot, with infuser or strainer, makes it easy to enjoy freshly brewed tea. Or you might do as "milady" did centuries ago and simply rest a tea strainer on the cup and pour the tea through it (as shown in Figure 5).

Figure 5. Pouring Tea Through a Strainer

The brewing of fine tea is best done in china, glass, or stainless steel. Never steep tea in plastic or aluminum. Don't use an aluminum kettle for boiling water for brewing tea either.

Always fill your teapot with hot water to preheat it. Empty it out only when the brewing water is ready.

PREPARING THE BREWING WATER

Always use fresh bottled water for brewing tea. Tap water contains chemicals that can alter the taste of a brew. Heat water for brewing to the temperatures suggested below, depending on the tea you are using. Never reheat water left in the kettle. Reheating water results in a flat cup of tea. It may seem terribly odd to be giving you directions for boiling water, but the correct steeping temperature is critical for certain teas, so please read on.

Green Teas and Light, Flowery Herbals

Steep in water that has not quite reached boiling (called the first boil). It's better to steep delicate teas a little longer using water at a lower temperature than it is to force the leaves to give up their essence with high temperatures and end up with a bitter brew.

Oolongs, Semi-Fermented Teas, and Most Herbal Blends

Steep in water at the second boil. This water is dancing and hissing with impatience. There are bubbles rising across the entire surface; it's starting to steam, on the verge of erupting. Water on the second boil will register between 180°F and 195°F.

Heavy Black Teas and Herbals with Roasted Ingredients

Steep in water at the third boil. Water at a full, rollicking boil is what's needed to release the full flavors of heavy traditional teas and hearty herb blends. You don't need a thermometer to identify water on the third boil.

When the brewing water is ready, empty the teapot and put a suitable amount of tea into it—one tea bag or one rounded teaspoon of loose tea per cup. Add boiling water, cover, and let steep for three to five minutes (three minutes for light flavor; five minutes for full rich flavor). Flavor increases with the length of the steeping period. Some teas produce color quickly, but don't be deceived. You can't judge when a tea is ready solely by color; take a test sip. Full flavor depends on at least three—preferably five—minutes of steeping time.

We predict that worldwide consumption of green tea will continue to increase as word spreads about its delicious flavor and the health benefits of the polyphenols in it. The amazing scientific research that we have summarized in this book is only the beginning; researchers are always learning more about green tea and how it promotes good health. More good news about green tea is sure to come in the coming months and years. Meanwhile, continue to enjoy green tea every day!

Glossary

ACQUIRED IMMUNODEFICIENCY SYNDROME (AIDS). A deadly, progressive disease caused by a virus, leading to compromised immune function.

AFLATOXIN. A carcinogen produced by molds, especially in stored agricultural crops, such as peanuts.

AGRANULOCYTOSIS. A rare condition in which the blood's content of granulocytes (a type of white blood cell) is drastically reduced, leading to compromised immune function.

ALZHEIMER'S DISEASE. A progressive brain disorder that gradually destroys a person's memory and ability to learn, reason, make judgments, communicate, and carry out daily activities.

AMINO ACIDS. The building blocks of protein.

ANEMIA. A condition characterized by a reduced number of red blood cells; symptoms include fatigue, unclear thinking, and poor concentration.

ANEURYSM. The localized enlargement of a blood vessel, forming a harmful bulge in the vessel wall.

Glossary

ANGINA PECTORIS. Sporadic chest pain caused by restricted blood flow to the heart, which decreases the oxygen supply to the heart muscle.

ANGIOGENESIS. The process of growing new blood vessels; it's valuable and important at times, but can also be used by cancerous tumors.

ANTIBODY. Any of a large number of proteins produced by the immune system that eliminate foreign substances present in the body.

ANTIOXIDANT. A substance that neutralizes free radicals otherwise associated with degenerative diseases, such as cancer, heart disease, and premature aging.

APOPTOSIS. Also called programmed cell death, this is a way for normal or cancerous cells to die.

AROMATIC OILS. Constituents of tea primarily responsible for its fragrance; also called volatile oils.

ARTERY. A blood vessel that carries blood from the heart to other tissues of the body.

ATHEROSCLEROSIS. A chronic disease in which fatty deposits of plaque restrict or block blood flow in the arteries; commonly known as "hardening of the arteries."

B CELL. A type of white blood cell that is part of the immune system and circulates in the blood on the alert for invading bacteria; also called B lymphocyte.

BACTERIA. Single-celled microorganisms; some cause disease, while others are harmless or even beneficial to biological processes.

BASAL METABOLIC RATE. The rate at which energy is used by a person at rest for maintaining basic body processes, such as breathing and the circulation of fluids.

BILE. A bitter fluid produced by the liver and stored in the gallbladder before being released into the small intestine to assist in the digestion of fats.

BLOOD PRESSURE. The forces placed on the blood vessels by the flow of blood.

BONE MARROW. The soft material that fills the inside of bone cavities and produces blood cells.

BOWEL. The small or large intestine.

CAFFEINE. An organic chemical present in tea. A member of the family of alkaloids, it acts as a stimulant to the central nervous system.

CAMELLIA SINENSIS. The Latin name for the tea plant.

CANCER. A general term for various illnesses characterized by abnormal growth of cells, leading to malignant tumors.

CAPILLARIES. Tiny blood vessels connecting the smallest arteries to the smallest veins.

CARBOHYDRATE. Any of various compounds of carbon, hydrogen, and oxygen—such as sugars, starches, and celluloses—produced by plants and bacteria and constituting an important part of the human diet.

CARCINOGEN. A potential cancer-causing agent.

CARDIOVASCULAR DISEASE. Any of the diseases affecting the heart and blood vessels, including coronary artery disease and hypertension.

CARIES. Decay of teeth due to bacteria; also known as tooth decay.

CARTILAGE. Dense connective tissue located in the joints, nose, and ears.

CATECHINS. Another name for the particular class of polyphenols found in green tea.

CAVITY. An area of a tooth where the enamel has been destroyed by bacterial action.

CEREBROVASCULAR DISEASE. A disease, such as stroke, that originates in the blood vessels of the brain.

CHAI. A mixture of black tea, milk, and spices that originated in India and is now popular worldwide.

CHANOYU. The Japanese tea ceremony; literally "hot water for tea."

CHEMOTHERAPY. Treatment of cancer using chemicals that are toxic to cancer cells.

CHOLESTEROL. A fat-like substance found in foods and produced by the liver. High levels circulating in the blood are a risk factor for cardiovascular disease.

CHRONIC RENAL FAILURE. Serious, long-term failure of the kidneys to function properly.

COLLAGEN. A protein that is the main component of connective tissues.

COLON. The large intestine extending from the small intestine to the anus.

CONSTIPATION. The difficult passage of hard, dry stools.

CORONARY ARTERY DISEASE. A cardiovascular disease specifically affecting the arteries that supply blood to the heart, often the cause of a heart attack.

CROHN'S DISEASE. Chronic, inflammatory condition of the gastrointestinal tract.

DEMENTIA. Mental deterioration leading to inability to think clearly or function normally.

DENTIN. The tissue of the tooth beneath the enamel and enclosing the pulp cavity.

DEOXYRIBONUCLEIC ACID (DNA). A substance found in the nucleus of cells that carries genetic information.

DETOXIFICATION. The process of cleansing the body of drugs and other toxins.

DIABETES. A disorder characterized by high levels of glucose in the blood. It may be caused by a failure of the pancreas to produce sufficient insulin or by resistance of the body to the action of insulin.

DUODENAL ULCER. An ulcer in the duodenum, the first or upper part of the small intestine.

EDEMA. Swelling of body tissues due to excessive fluid accumulation.

ELECTROLYTE. A substance, such as a salt, that dissolves into positively and negatively charged particles, the solution of which conducts an electrical charge. Sodium, potassium, and chloride are examples of the particles, and table salt and baking soda are examples of electrolytes.

ENAMEL. The hard, calcified outer layer of the teeth.

ENZYME. A complex protein present in digestive juices or within cells that acts as a catalyst for chemical reactions.

ERGOGENIC AID. Any substance that improves athletic performance.

ESOPHAGUS. The muscular tube that connects the throat to the stomach.

ESTROGEN. A hormone produced primarily in women that stimulates the development of female secondary sex characteristics and contributes to cyclical changes, such as menstruation and menopause.

FECES. Bodily waste discharged from the bowels.

FIBRINOGEN. A protein in the blood involved in the clotting process.

FIBROCYSTIC BREAST DISEASE. An umbrella term for any condition of the breasts characterized by painful lumps.

FLAVONOID. A phytonutrient, composed of particular arrangements of carbon, hydrogen, and oxygen atoms, that frequently has antioxidant, disease-preventing effects.

FREE RADICAL. A highly reactive compound that damages cell membranes and other cell components, contributing to degenerative diseases, such as heart disease, cancer, premature aging, cataracts, and arthritis. Free radicals are found in air pollution, tobacco smoke, some foods, and pesticides. Some are produced by ultraviolet radiation; they are also manufactured during normal body processes. Chemically, free radicals have single, unshared electrons that are responsible for their high reactivity.

FRENCH PARADOX. The unusual phenomenon of a low rate of heart disease in a country where the typical diet is high in fat.

GALLBLADDER. A sac located under the liver that stores bile secreted from the liver.

GAP JUNCTION. A pore in cell membranes, through which cells communicate with one another by transferring substances.

GASTROINTESTINAL TRACT. The digestive system, including the stomach and the intestines.

GINGIVITIS. Inflammation of the dental gums, the beginning stage of periodontal disease.

GLUCOSE. A particular sugar that occurs widely in nature. The term is often used to refer to the sugar commonly found in the blood, in which case it is a synonym for blood sugar.

GLYCOGEN. A carbohydrate polymer composed of glucose units. It is the main form in which carbohydrate is stored in the body. The liver produces glycogen from glucose and stores it until the muscles need it for energy.

GRAM-NEGATIVE BACTERIA. A class of bacteria, including the common bacterium *E. coli*, that stain pink in a laboratory diagnostic procedure that was developed by Danish physician Hans C. J. Gram.

GRAM-POSITIVE BACTERIA. A class of bacteria, including the bacterium that causes botulism, that stain blue in a laboratory diagnostic procedure that was developed by Danish physician Hans C. J. Gram.

GRANULOCYTE. A type of white blood cell.

HDL-CHOLESTEROL. High-density lipoprotein cholesterol that transports fats in the blood for removal. Within recommended limits for blood cholesterol overall, a high level of HDL-cholesterol relative to LDL-cholesterol is associated with a reduced risk of heart disease.

HEART ATTACK. A condition involving serious organ damage that occurs when the blood flow to the heart is severely limited or stopped; also called myocardial infarction.

HOMOCYSTEINE. Amino acid–like compound; elevated levels increase the risk of cardiovascular disease.

HPV (HUMAN PAPILLOMAVIRUS). More than one hundred different viruses are in this family; some cause genital warts and other increase the chances of cervical cancer.

HUMAN IMMUNODEFICIENCY VIRUS (HIV). The virus that causes AIDS.

HYPERTENSION. High blood pressure. Blood pressure readings above 140/90 are considered high and indicate that the heart and arteries are under excessive strain.

HYPERTHYROIDISM. A condition in which the thyroid gland produces excessive amounts of thyroid hormone.

IMMUNE SYSTEM. The system that protects the body from disease. It consists of many specialized organs, tissues, and chemicals that work together, including the spleen, lymph nodes, and white blood cells.

INFLAMMATORY BOWEL DISEASE. Group of inflammatory conditions afflicting the large intestine, including Crohn's disease and ulcerative colitis.

INFLUENZA. A viral infection causing symptoms similar to the common cold, which can lead to serious complications.

INSULIN. A hormone produced by the pancreas that regulates blood sugar levels.

INTERFERON. A protein produced by the immune system that inhibits a virus from infecting cells.

KIDNEYS. The two bean-shaped organs responsible for the excretion of urine and regulation of water and electrolyte levels in the body.

LDL-CHOLESTEROL. Low-density lipoprotein cholesterol that transports fats within the bloodstream; it is known as the "bad" cholesterol because high levels of LDL-cholesterol are associated with an increased risk of heart disease.

LEUKOCYTE. Any of the white blood cells.

LIVER. An important organ that secretes bile, detoxifies the blood, and stores glycogen.

L-THEANINE. Amino acid unique to green tea; it contributes to taste and has been shown to convey a sense of calm.

LYMPHOCYTE. A specialized white blood cell that aids the body in the protection against disease and infection. They are further divided into B cells and T cells.

METASTASIS. The spread of a cancer from the original site to another part of the body.

METHYLXANTHINE. Any of a group of related compounds, including caffeine, theobromine, and theophylline.

MICROORGANISMS. Bacteria, viruses, fungi, and other minute life forms that are only visible through a microscope; many of these cause infections.

MINERAL. An inorganic substance. Many are nutrients essential for the growth, maintenance, and repair of the human body.

MITOCHONDRIA. Any of various specialized structures found in all cells that are responsible for producing energy for the cell.

MUTAGEN. A substance that causes a genetic mutation, possibly predisposing a cell to cancer development.

NEUROTRANSMITTER. Any of several chemical substances that transmit impulses from one nerve cell to another or from a nerve cell to a muscle or gland.

OBESITY. A condition in which the body stores excessive amounts of fat. Body weight in excess of 20 percent above ideal body weight is considered obese.

ORAL. Pertaining to the mouth.

OSTEOGENESIS IMPERFECTA. A rare inherited disease in which the bones are abnormally brittle and fragile.

OSTEOPOROSIS. A condition characterized by porous, brittle bones that are prone to fractures.

OXIDATION. A process in which one or more electrons are removed from an atom or molecule, especially as a part of the process of free radical damage to cells, tissues, and organs that is associated with an increased risk of heart disease, cancer, and other degenerative diseases.

PANCREAS. An organ in the abdomen responsible for producing and secreting several digestive enzymes and the hormone insulin.

PARKINSON'S DISEASE. Degenerative disorder of the central nervous system that can impair motor skills and speech.

PERIODONTAL DISEASE. A serious dental condition in which the gums are inflamed and may recede from the tooth, and teeth may loosen.

PH. A measure of the acidity and alkalinity of a solution.

PHYTONUTRIENT. Chemical compounds, found in plants (*phyto* is derived from the Greek word for plant), that have health benefits but are not (despite the name) nutrients.

PLACEBO. An inactive substance used in controlled experiments that is intended to test the effects of another substance.

PLAQUE. (1) A deposit of bacteria and other material that can build up on the tooth surfaces and lead to tooth decay. (2) Deposits of cholesterol that build up along blood vessel walls.

PLATELET. One of the small, round, disk-shaped blood cells necessary for clotting.

POLYPHENOLS. Naturally occurring compounds, composed of carbon, hydrogen, and oxygen atoms in particular arrangements, that are powerful antioxidants. The four primary polyphenols in green tea are epicatechin (EC), epicatechin gallate (ECG), epigallocatechin (EGC), and epigallocatechin gallate (EGCG). They serve a protective role because they are very easily oxidized in preference to other molecules in their vicinity.

PREMENSTRUAL SYNDROME. A combination of physical and emotional symptoms occurring a week or two before menstruation.

PROSTATE GLAND. A gland located at the base of the bladder in men.

RADIATION THERAPY. A cancer treatment in which X-rays or gamma rays are targeted at a tumor.

RED TEA. Sometimes called Rooibos, this tisane is made from the needle-like leaves of a South African shrub. Similar in taste to black tea; it also has antioxidant and cancer-preventive properties.

SAMOVAR. A metal urn with a spigot used to boil water for tea.

SCURVY. A disease caused by a deficiency of vitamin C, resulting in bleeding gums, loose teeth, bruising, and weakness.

SICKLE CELL ANEMIA. Genetic disorder that adversely affects red blood cells.

STREPTOCOCCUS MUTANS. The bacterium responsible for the development of dental plaque.

STROKE. Brain damage caused by a ruptured or blocked blood vessel in the brain.

T CELL. A type of white blood cell that patrols the body for foreign matter and cancer cells.

THROMBOXANE. A fatty acid derivative that initiates the blood clotting process.

THYMUS GLAND. A gland in the chest that participates in the production of particular white blood cells.

TISANE. Correct name for an infusion of herbs in hot water that is consumed in a way similar to drinking tea.

TUMOR. An abnormal growth of tissue, which may be cancerous (malignant) or noncancerous (benign).

ULCERATIVE COLITIS. A form of inflammatory bowel disease and a cause of diarrhea.

ULTRAVIOLET RADIATION. Radiation similar to visible light, but having wavelengths shorter than visible light. The body uses ultraviolet radiation to produce vitamin D. Ultraviolet radiation also causes sunburn and can create free radicals.

VIRUS. A tiny subcellular organism that causes disease.

VITAMIN. A nutrient that is absolutely essential to the body but of which only minute quantities are required.

Notes

INTRODUCTION: GREEN TEA AND ITS HEALTH BENEFITS

1. Gardner, E. J., Ruxton, C. H., and Leeds, A. R. Black tea—helpful or harmful? A review of the evidence. *European Journal of Clinical Nutrition.* 61:3–18, 2007.
2. Lin, Y. L., Juan, I. M., Chen, Y. L., et al. Composition of polyphenols in fresh tea leaves and associations of their oxygen-radical-absorbing capacity with antiproliferative actions in fibroblast cells. *Journal of Agricultural and Food Chemistry.* 44(6):1387–1394, 1996.

CHAPTER 1. A MEDICINE CHEST OF GOOD HEALTH

1. Kono, S., Shinchi, K., Ikeda, N., et al. Green tea consumption and serum lipid profiles: a cross-sectional study in Northern Kyushu, Japan. *Preventive Medicine.* 21:526–531, 1992.
2. Yamaguchi, Y., Hayashi, M., Yamazoe, H., et al. Preventive effects of green tea extract on lipid abnormalities in serum, liver, and aorta of mice fed an atherogenic diet. *Nippon Ronen Igakkai Zasshi (Japanese Journal of Geriatrics).* 97(6):329–337, 1991.
3. Sagesaka-Mitane, Y., Milwa, M., and Okada, S. Platelet aggregation inhibitors in hot water extract of green tea. *Chemical & Pharmaceutical Bulletin.* 38(3):790–793, 1990.
4. Stensvold, I., Tverdal, A., Solvoll, K., et al. Tea consumption. Relationship to cholesterol, blood pressure, and coronary and total mortality. *Preventive Medicine.* 21:546–553, 1992.
5. Gao, Y. T., McLaughlin, J. K., Blot, W. J., at al. Reduced risk of esophageal cancer associated with green tea consumption. *Journal of the National Cancer Institute.* 86(11):855–858, 1994.

   Narisawa, T., and Fukaura, Y. A very low dose of green tea polyphenols in drinking water prevents N-methyl-N-nitrosourea-induced colon carcinogenesis. *Japanese Journal of Cancer Research.* 84:1007–1009, 1993.

   Ohno, Y., Wakai, K., Genka, K., et al. Tea consumption and lung cancer risk: a case-control study in Okinawa, Japan. *Japanese Journal of Cancer Research.* 86:1027–1034, 1995.

Liao, S., Umekita, Y., Guo, J., et al. Growth inhibition and regression of human prostate and breast tumors in athymic mice by tea epigallocatechin gallate. *Cancer Letters.* 96:239–243, 1995.

Stoner, G. D., and Mukhtar, H. Polyphenols as cancer chemopreventive agents. *Journal of Cellular Biochemistry.* 22:169–180, 1995.

6. Morre, D. J., Morre, D. M., Sun, H., et al. Tea catechin synergies in inhibition of cancer cell proliferation and of a cancer specific cell surface oxidase (ECTO-NOX). *Pharmacology and Toxicology.* 92:234–241, 2003.

7. Zheng, W., Doyle, T. J., Kushi, L. H., et al. Tea consumption and cancer incidence in a prospective cohort study of postmenopausal women. *American Journal of Epidemiology.* 144(2):175–182, 1996.

8. Sadakata, S., Fukao, A., and Hisamichi, S. Mortality among female practitioners of chanoyu (Japanese "tea-ceremony"). *Tohoku Journal of Experimental Medicine.* 166(4):475–477, 1992.

9. Ikigai, H., Nakae, T., Hara, Y., et al. Bactericidal catechins damage the lipid bilayer. *Biochimia et Biophysica Acta.* 1147:132–136, 1993.

Hamilton-Miller, J. M. Antimicrobial properties of tea (*Camellia sinensis* L.). *Antimicrobial Agents and Chemotherapy.* 39(11):2375–2377, 1995.

Toda, M., Okubo, S., Ohnishi, R., et al. Antibacterial and bactericidal activities of Japanese green tea. *Japanese Journal of Bacteriology.* 44(4):669–672, 1989.

Nakayama, M., Suzuki, K., Toda, M., et al. Inhibition of the infectivity of influenza virus by tea polyphenols. *Antiviral Research.* 21:289–299, 1993.

10. Ooshima, T., Minami, T., Aono, W., et al. Oolong tea polyphenols inhibit experimental dental caries in SPF rats infected with mutans streptococci. *Caries Research.* 27(2):124–129, 1993.

Ooshima, T., Minami, T., Aono, W., et al. Reduction of dental plaque deposition in humans by oolong tea extract. *Caries Research.* 28(3):146–149, 1994.

11. Yang, C. S., and Wang, Z. Tea and cancer. *Journal of the National Cancer Institute.* 85(13):1038–1049, 1993.

12. Miura, S., Watanabe, J., Sano, M., et al. Effects of various antioxidants on the Cu (2+)-mediated oxidative modification of low density lipoprotein. *Biological & Pharmaceutical Bulletin.* 18(1):1–4, 1995.

13. Graham, H. N. Green tea composition, consumption, and polyphenol chemistry. *Preventive Medicine* 21:334–350, 1992.

14. Ho, C., Chen, Q., Shi, H., et al. Antioxidative effect of polyphenol extract prepared from various Chinese teas. *Preventive Medicine.* 21:520–525, 1992.

15. Gilbert, R. M. Caffeine consumption. *Progress in Clinical & Biological Research.* 158:185–213, 1984.

16. Jarvis, M. J. Does caffeine intake enhance absolute levels of cognitive performance? *Psychopharmacology.* 110(1–2):45–52, 1993.

17. Lamarine, R. J. Selected health and behavioral effects related to the use of caffeine. *Journal of Community Health.* 19(6):449–467, December 1994.

18. Gardner, E. J., Ruxton, C. H., and Leeds, A. R. Black tea—helpful or harmful? A review of the evidence. *European Journal of Clinical Nutrition.* 61:3–18, 2007.

19. Ma, Y. H., Recknagel, S., Bratter, P., et al. Determination of minerals and trace elements in selenium tea from the Enschi district, People's Republic of China, and in its infusions using inductively coupled plasma-atomic emission spectrometry, graphite furnace atomic absorption spectrometry, and instrumental

neutron activation analysis. *Zeitschrift fur Lebensmittel Untersuchung und Forschung.* 197(5):444–448, November 1993.

Wenlock, R. W., Buss, D. H., and Dixon, E. J. Trace nutrients. Manganese in British food. *British Journal of Nutrition.* 41(2):253–261, March 1979.

20. Asanami, S., Tanabe, Y., Koga, H., et al. Fluoride contents in tea and Sakura-shrimp in relation to other inorganic constituents. *Shoni Shikagaku Zasshi (Japanese Journal of Pedodontics).* 89(8):1407–1412, August 1989.

21. Fukushima, M., and Tanimura, A. Action and absorption possibility of aluminium in infused green tea, black tea, oolong tea, and instant coffee solution at simulated human gastric juice. *Journal of the Japanese Society for Food Science & Technology—Nippon.* 43(8):939–945, 1996.

Drewitt, P. N., Butterworth, K. R., Springall, C. D., et al. Plasma levels of aluminium after tea ingestion in healthy volunteers. *Food and Chemical Toxicology.* 31(1):19–23, January 1993.

22. Ito, K., Nagato, Y., Aoi, N., et al. Effects of L-theanine on the release of alpha-brain waves in human volunteers. *Nippon Nogeikagaku Kaishi.* 72:153–157, 1998.

CHAPTER 2. THE "HOTTEST" HISTORIC BEVERAGE

Works Consulted:

Baker, William. *Running Her Fasting Down.* Caldwell, Idaho: Caxton, 1974.

Kakuzo, Okakura. *The Book of Tea.* Rutland, Vermont: Charles E. Tuttle, 1956.

Perry, Sara. *The Tea Book.* San Francisco: Chronicle Books, 1993.

Pratt, James Norwood. *Tea Lover's Treasury.* Santa Rosa, Calif.: Cole Group, 1982.

Scharpira, Joel, Scharpira, David, and Scharpira, Karl. *The Book of Coffee & Tea.* New York: St. Martin's Press, 1975.

San, Soshitsu. *Chado: The Japanese Way of Tea.* New York: John Weatherhill, 1979.

Sadler, Arthur. *Cha-no-yu The Japanese Tea Ceremony.* Rutland, Vermont: Charles E. Tuttle, 1962.

Tanaka, Sen'o. *The Tea Ceremony.* New York: Harmony Books, 1973.

CHAPTER 3. ANTIOXIDANTS

1. Ames, B. N., Shigenaga, M. K., Hagen, T. M. Oxidants, antioxidants, and the degenerative diseases of aging. *Proceedings of the National Academy of Sciences, U. S. A.* 90:7915–7922, 1993.

2. Cao, G. H., Sofic, E., and Prior, R. L. Antioxidant capacity of tea and common vegetables. *Journal of Agricultural and Food Chemistry.* 44(11):3426–3431, 1996.

3. Hertog, M. G., Hollman, P. C., Katan, M. D., et al. Intake of potentially anti-carcinogenic flavonoids and their determinants in adults in The Netherlands, *Nutrition and Cancer.* 20(1):21–29, 1993.

4. Hertog, M. G., Feskens, E. J., Hollman, P. C., et al. Dietary antioxidant flavonoids and risk of coronary heart disease: The Zutphen Elderly Study. *Lancet* 342(8878):1007–1011, 1993.

5. Hertog, M. G., Kromhout, D., Aravanis, C., et al. Flavonoid intake and long-term risk of coronary heart disease and cancer in the Seven Countries Study. *Archives of Internal Medicine.* 155:381–386, 1995.

6. Keli, S. O., Hertog, M. G., Feskens, E. J., et al. Dietary flavonoids, antioxidant vitamins, and incidence of stroke. *Archives of Internal Medicine.* 156:637–642, 1996.

7. Rice-Evans, C. A., Miller, N. J., and Paganga, G. Structure-antioxidant activity

relationships of flavonoids and phenolic acids. *Free Radical Biology & Medicine.* 20(7):933–956, 1996.

8. Nanjo, F., Goto, K., Seto, R., et al. Scavenging effects of tea catechins and their derivatives on 1,1-diphenyl-2-picrylhydrazyl radical. *Free Radical Biology & Medicine.* 21(6):895–902, 1996.

9. Salah, N., Miller, N. J., Paganga, G., et al. Polyphenolic flavonols as scavengers of aqueous phase radicals and as chain-breaking antioxidants. *Archives of Biochemistry & Biophysics.* 322(2):339–346, 1995.

10. Nanjo, F., Honda, M., Okushio, K., et al. Effects of dietary tea catechins on alpha-tocopherol levels, lipid peroxidation, and erythrocyte deformability in rats fed on high palm oil and perilla oil diets. *Biological & Pharmaceutical Bulletin.* 16(11):1156–1159, 1993.

11. Maxwell, S., and Thorpe, G. Tea flavonoids have little short term impact on serum antioxidant activity. *British Medical Journal.* 313(7051):229, 1996.

    Shiraki, M., Hara, Y., Osawa, T., et al. Antioxidative and antimutagenic effects of theaflavins from black tea. *Mutation Research.* 323:29–34, 1994.

    Miller, N. J., Castelluccio, C., Tijburg, L., et al. The antioxidant properties of theaflavins and their gallate esters: radical scavengers or metal chelators? *FEBS Letters.* 392:40–44, 1996.

12. Ho, C., Chen, Q., Shi, H., et al. Antioxidative effect of polyphenol extract prepared from various Chinese teas. *Preventive Medicine* 21:520–525, 1992.

13. He, Y. H., and Kies, C. Green and black tea consumption by humans. Impact on polyphenol concentration in feces, blood, and urine. *Plant Foods for Human Nutrition.* 46(3):221–229, 1994.

14. Gardner, E. J., Ruxton, C. H., and Leeds, A. R. Black tea—helpful or harmful? A review of the evidence. *European Journal of Clinical Nutrition.* 61:3–18, 2007.

15. Serafini, M., Ghiselli, A., and Ferro-Luzzi, A. *In vivo* antioxidant effect of green and black tea in man. *European Journal of Clinical Nutrition.* 50(1):28–32, 1996.

    Serafini, M., Ghiselli, A., and Ferro-Luzzi, A. Red wine, tea, and antioxidants. *Lancet.* 344:626, 1994.

16. Wu., Y. Scavenging action of green tea extract on singlet oxygen and preventive effect on lipid peroxidation. *Chung Hua Kou Chiang i Hsueh Tsa Chih Chinese Journal of Stomatology.* 15(5):354–359, 1993.

    Ruth, R. J., Cheng, S. J., and Klaunig, J. E. Prevention of cytotoxicity and inhibition of intercellular communication by antioxidant catechins isolated from Chinese green tea. *Carcinogenesis.* 10(6):1003–1008, 1989.

17. Pingzhang, Y., Jinying, Z., Shujun, C., et al. Experimental studies of the inhibitory effects of green tea catechin on mice large intestinal cancers induced by 1,2-dimethylhydrazine. *Cancer Letters.* 79:33–38, 1994.

    Khan, S. G., Katiyar, S. K., Agarwal, R., et al. Enhancement of antioxidant and phase II enzymes by oral feeding of green tea polyphenols in drinking water to SKH-1 hairless mice. Possible role in cancer chemoprevention. *Cancer Research.* 52:4050–4052, 1992.

CHAPTER 4. CANCER PREVENTION IN THE TEAPOT

1. Zheng, W., Doyle, T. J., Kushi, L. H., et al. Tea consumption and cancer incidence in a prospective cohort study of postmenopausal women. *American Journal of Epidemiology.* 144:175–182, 1996.

2. Valcic, S., Timmermann, B. N., Alberts, D. S., et al. Inhibitory effect of six green

tea catechins and caffeine on the growth of four selected human tumor cell lines. *Anti-Cancer Drugs.* 7(4):461–468, 1996.

Apostolides, Z., and Weisburger, J. H. Screening of tea clones for inhibition of PhIP mutagenicity. *Mutation Research.* 326:219–225, 1995.

3. Smith, T. J., Hong, J., Wang, Z., et al. How can carcinogenesis be inhibited? *Annals of the New York Academy of Sciences.* 768:82–90, September 30, 1995.

4. Khan, S. G., Katiyar, S. K., Agarwal, R., et al. Enhancement of antioxidant and phase II enzymes by oral feeding of green tea polyphenols in drinking water to SKH-1 hairless mice. Possible role in cancer chemoprevention. *Cancer Research.* 52:4050–1052, 1992.

5. Wang, H., and Wu, Y. Inhibitory effect of Chinese tea on N-nitrosation *in vitro* and *in vivo*. *IARC Scientific Publications.* 105:546–549, 1991.

Yan, Y. S. The experiment of tumor-inhibiting effect of green tea extract in animal and human body. *Chinese Journal of Preventive Medicine.* 27(3):129–131, May 1993.

6. Bu-Abbas, A., Clifford, M. N., Ioannides, C., et al. Stimulation of rat hepatic UDP-glucuronosyl transferase activity following treatment with green tea. *Food and Chemical Toxicology.* 33(1):27–30, January 1995.

7. Liu, L., and Castonguay, A. Inhibition of the metabolism and genotoxicity of 4-(methylnitrosamino)-1-(3-pyridyl)-1-butanone (NNK) in rat hepatocytes by (+)-catechin. *Carcinogenesis.* 12(7):1203–1208, July 1991.

Yen, G. C., and Chen, H. Y. Relationship between antimutagenic activity and major components of various teas. *Mutagenesis.* 11(1):37–41, January 1996.

Kada, T., Kaneko, K., Matsuzaki, S., et al. Detection and chemical identification of natural bioantimutagens. A case of the green tea factor. *Mutation Research.* 150(1–2):127–132, 1985.

8. Sasaki, Y. F., Yamada, H., Shimoi, K., et al. The clastogen-suppressing effects of green tea, Po-lei tea and Rooibos tea in CHO cells and mice. *Mutation Research.* 286:221–232, 1993.

9. Hayatsu, H., Inada, N., Kakutani, T., et al. Suppression of genotoxicity of carcinogens by (−)-epigallocatechin gallate. *Preventive Medicine* 21:370–376, 1992.

10. Ruch, R. J., Cheng, S. J., and Klaunig, J. E. Prevention of cytotoxicity and inhibition of intercellular communication by antioxidant catechins isolated from Chinese green tea. *Carcinogenesis.* 10(6):1003–1008, June 1989.

11. Hou, Z., Lambert, J. D., Chin, K. V., et al. Effects of tea polyphenols on signal transduction pathways related to cancer chemoprevention. *Mutatation Research.* 555(1–2):3–19, 2004.

12. Hu, G., and Chen, J. Inhibition of oncogene expression by green tea and (−)-epigallocatechin gallate in mice. *Nutrition and Cancer.* 24:203–209, 1995.

Wadatani, M., Ohtani, K., Kageyama, K., et al. Prevention of ornithine decarboxylase induction in Ehrlick ascites tumor cells by tea polyphenols. *Cancer Journal.* 9(3):161–167, 1996.

13. Mukhtar, H., Wang, Z. Y., Katiyar, S. K., et al. Tea components. Antimutagenic and anticarcinogenic effects. *Preventive Medicine.* 21:351–360, 1992.

14. Isemura, M., Saeki, K., Kimura, T., et al. Tea catechins and related polyphenols as anti-cancer agents. *Biofactors.* 13(1–4):81–85, 2000.

Kuo, P. L., and Lin, C. C. Green tea constituent (−)-epigallocatechin-3-gallate inhibits Hep G2 cell proliferation and induces apoptosis through p53-dependent and Fas-mediated pathways. *Journal of Biomedical Sciences.* 10(2):219–227, 2003.

15. Fujiki, H., Yoshizawa, S., Horiuchi, T., et al. Anticarcinogenic effects of (-)-epigallocatechin gallate. *Preventive Medicine.* 21:503–509, 1992.

CHAPTER 5. TEA'S EFFECT ON CANCERS AND SIDE EFFECTS OF CANCER TREATMENTS

1. Katiyar, S. K., Agarwal, R, Wood, G. S., et al. Inhibition of 12-o-tetradecanoyl-phorbol-13-acetate-caused tumor promotion in 7,12-dimethylbenz[a]anthracene-initiated SENCAR mouse skin by a polyphenolic fraction isolated from green tea. *Cancer Research.* 52:6890–6897, 1992.

   Katiyar, S. K., Agarwal, R., and Mukhtar, H. Inhibition of both stage I and stage II skin tumor promotion in SENCAR mice by a polyphenolic fraction isolated from green tea. Inhibition depends on the duration of polyphenol treatment. *Carcinogenesis.* 14(12):2641–2643, 1993.

   Katiyar, S. K., Agarwal, R., Ekker, S., et al. Protection against 12-O-tetrade-canoylphorbol-13-acetate-caused inflammation in SENCAR mouse ear skin by polyphenolic fraction isolated from green tea. *Carcinogenesis.* 14(3):361–365, 1993.

   Katiyar, S. K., Elmets, C. A., Agarwal, R., et al. Protection against ultraviolet-B radiation-induced local and systemic suppression of contact hypersensitivity and edema responses in C3H/HeN mice by green tea polyphenols. *Photochemistry & Photobiology.* 62(5):855–861, 1995.

   Katiyar, S. K., Agarwal, R., and Mukhtar, H. Protection against malignant conversion of chemically induced benign skin, papillomas to squamous cell carcinomas in SENCAR mice by a polyphenolic fraction isolated from green tea. *Cancer Research.* 53:5409–5412, 1993.

   Baba, N., Shinmoto, H., Kobori, M., et al. Effects of some edible plants on melanin production, immunoglobulin secretion and differentiation of cultured mammalian cell lines. *Journal of the Japanese Society for Food Science & Technology—Nippon.* 43(5):622–628, 1996.

2. Hakim, I. A., Harris, R. B., and Weisgerber, U. M. Tea intake and squamous cell carcinoma of the skin: influence of type of tea beverages. *Cancer Epidemiology, Biomarkers, and Prevention.* 9(7):727–731, 2000.

   Katiyar, S. K., Perez, A., and Mukhtar, H. Green tea polyphenol treatment to human skin prevents formation of ultraviolet light B-induced pyrimidine dimers in DNA. *Clinical Cancer Research.* 6(10):3864–3869, 2000.

   Katiyar, S., Elmets, C. A., and Katiyar, S. K. Green tea and skin cancer: photoimmunology, angiogenesis and DNA repair. *Journal of Nutritional Biochemistry.* 18(5):287–96, 2006.

3. Yang, C. S., and Wang, Z. Tea and cancer. *Journal of the National Cancer Institute.* 85(13):1038–1049, 1993.

   Dhar, G. M., Shah, G. N., Naheed, B., et al. Epidemiological trend in the distribution of cancer in Kashmir Valley. *Journal of Epidemiology & Community Health.* 47(4):290–292, 1993.

4. Chen, J. The effects of Chinese tea on the occurrence of esophageal tumors induced by N-nitrosomethylbenzylamine in rats. *Preventive Medicine.* 21:385–391, 1992.

5. Wang, Z. Y, Wang, L., Lee, M., et al. Inhibition of N-nitrosomethylbenzylamine-induced esophageal tumorigenesis in rats by green and black tea. *Carcinogenesis.* 16(9):2143–2148, 1995.

6. Gao, Y. T., McLaughlin, J. K., Blot, W. J., et al. Reduced risk of esophageal cancer associated with green tea consumption. *Journal of the National Cancer Institute.* 86(11):855–858, 1994.

7. Li, N., Zheng, S., Han, C., and Chen, J. The chemoprotective effects of tea on human oral precancerous mucosa lesions. *Proceedings of the Society of Experimental Biological Medicine.* 220:218–224, 1999.

Li, N., Chen, X., Liao, J., et al. Inhibition of 7,12-dimethylbenz[a]anthracene (DMBA)-induced oral carcinogenesis in hamsters by tea and curcumin. *Carcinogenesis.* 23(8):1307–1313, 2002.

8. Hoshiyama, Y., Kawaguchi, T., Miura, Y., et al. A nested case-control study of stomach cancer in relation to green tea consumption in Japan. *British Journal of Cancer.* 90(1):135–138, 2004.

Koizumi, Y., Tsubono, Y., Nakaya, N., et al. No association between green tea and the risk of gastric cancer: pooled analysis of two prospective studies in Japan. *Cancer Epidemiology, Biomarkers, and Prevention.* 12(5):472–473, 2003.

Sun, C. L., Yuan, J. M., Lee, M. J., et al. Urinary tea polyphenols in relation to gastric and esophageal cancers: a prospective study of men in Shanghai, China. *Carcinogenesis.* 23(9):1497–1503, 2002.

9. Kona, S., Ikeda, M., Tokudome, S., et al. A case-control study of gastric cancer and diet in northern Kyushu, Japan. *Japanese Journal of Cancer Research.* 79:1067–1074, 1988.

Yu, G. P., Hsieh, C. C., Wang, L. Y., et al. Green tea consumption and risk of stomach cancer. A population-based case-control study in Shanghai, China. *Cancer Causes & Control.* 6(6):532–538, 1995.

Ji, B., Chow, W., Yang, G., et al. The influence of cigarette smoking, alcohol, and green tea consumption on the risk of carcinoma of the cardia and distal stomach in Shanghai, China. *Cancer.* 77:2449–2457, 1996.

Stich, H. F. Teas and tea consumption as inhibitors of carcinogen formation in model systems and man. *Preventive Medicine.* 21:377–384, 1992.

10. Hirose, M., Hoshiya, T., Akagi, K., et al. Effects of green tea catechins in a rat multi-organ carcinogenesis model. *Carcinogenesis.* 14(8):1549–1553, 1993.

Yamane, T., Nakatani, H., Kikuoka, N., et al. Inhibitory effects and toxicity of green tea polyphenols for gastrointestinal carcinogenesis. *Cancer.* 77:1662–1667, 1996.

Pingzhang, Y., Jinying, Z., Shujun, C., et al. Experimental studies of the inhibitory effects of green tea catechin on mice large intestinal cancers induced by 1,2-dimethylhydrazine. *Cancer Letters.* 79:33038, 1994.

11. Dora, I., Arab, L., Martinchik, A., et al. Black tea consumption and risk of rectal cancer in Moscow population. *Annals of Epidemiology.* 13(6):405–411, 2003.

Su, L. J., and Arab, L. Tea consumption and the reduced risk of colon cancer—results from a national prospective cohort study. *Public Health Nutrition.* 5(3):419–425, 2002.

12. Xu, M., Bailey, A. C., Hernaez, J. F., et al. Protection by green tea, black tea, and indole-3-carbinol against 2-amino-methylimidazo[4,5-f]quinoline-induced DNA adducts and colonic aberrant crypts in the F344 rat. *Carcinogenesis.* 17(7):1429–1434, 1996.

Inagake, M., Yamane, T., Kitao, Y., et al. Inhibition of 1,2-dimethylhydrazine-induced oxidative DNA damage by green tea extract in rat. *Japanese Journal of Cancer Research.* 86:1106–1111, 1995.

Narisawa, T., and Fukaura, Y. A very low dose of green tea polyphenols in drinking water prevents N-methyl-N-nitrosourea-induced colon carcinogenesis in F344 rats. *Japanese Journal of Cancer Research.* 84:1007–1009, 1993.

Yamane, I, Hagiwara, N., Tateishi, M., et al. Inhibition of azoxymethane-induced colon carcinogenesis in rat by green tea polyphenol fraction. *Japanese Journal of Cancer Research.* 82(12):1336–1339, 1991.

Kono, S., Shinchi, K., Ikeda, N., et al. Physical activity, dietary habits and adenomatous polyps of the sigmoid colon. A study of self-defense officials in Japan. *Journal of Clinical Epidemiology.* 44(11):1255–1261, 1991.

13. Arts, I. C., Jacobs, D. R., Jr., Gross, M., et al. Dietary catechins and cancer incidence among postmenopausal women: the Iowa Women's Health Study (United States). *Cancer Causes Control.* 13(4):373–382, 2002.

Ji, B. T., Chow, W. H., Hsing, A. W., et al. Green tea consumption and the risk of pancreatic and colorectal cancers. *International Journal of Cancer.* 70(3):255–258, 1997.

14. Wang, Z. Y., Agarwal, R., Khan, W., et al. Protection against benzo-[a]pyrene- and N-nitrosodiethylamine-induced lung and forestomach tumorigenesis in A/J mice by water extracts of green tea and licorice. *Carcinogenesis.* 13(8):1491–1494, 1992.

Sazuka, M., Murakami, S., Isemura, M., et al. Inhibitory effects of green tea infusion on *in vitro* invasion and *in vivo* metastasis of mouse lung carcinoma cells. *Cancer Letters.* 98:27–31, 1995.

Luo, D., and Li, Y. Preventive effect of green tea on MNNG-induced lung cancers and precancerous lesions in LACA mice. *Journal of West China University Medical Sciences.* 23(4):433–437, 1992.

15. Ohno, Y., Wakai, K., Genka, K., et al. Tea consumption and lung cancer risk. A case-control study in Okinawa, Japan. *Japanese Journal of Cancer Research.* 86:1027–1034, 1995.

16. Xu, Y., Ho, C., Amin, S. G., et al. Inhibition of tobacco-specific nitrosamine-induced lung tumorigenesis in A/J mice by green tea and its major polyphenol as antioxidants. *Cancer Research.* 52:3875–3879, 1992.

Shi, S. T., Wang, Z., Smith, T. J., et al. Effects of green tea and black tea on 4-(methylnitrosamino)-1-(3-pyridyl)-1-butanone bioactivation, DNA methylation, and lung tumorigenesis in A/J mice. *Cancer Research.* 54:4641–4647, 1994.

17. Shim, J. S., Kang, M. H., Kim, Y. H., et al. Chemopreventive effect of green tea (*Camellia sinensis*) among cigarette smokers. *Cancer Epidemiology, Biomarkers & Prevention.* 4(4):387–391, 1995.

18. Lee, A. H., Fraser, M. L., Meng, X., et al. Protective effects of green tea against prostate cancer. *Expert Review of Anticancer Therapy.* 6(4):507–513, 2006.

19. Severson, R. K., et al. A prospective study of demographics, diet, and prostate cancer among men of Japanese ancestry in Hawaii. *Cancer Research.* 49:1857–1860, 1989.

20. Yatani, R., et al. Geographic pathology of latent prostatic carcinoma. *International Journal of Cancer.* 29(6):611–616, 1982.

21. Liao, S., Umekita, Y., Guo J., et al. Growth inhibition and regression of human prostate and breast tumors in athymic mice by tea epigallocatechin gallate. *Cancer Research.* 96:239–243, 1995.

22. Bettuzzi, S., Brausi, M., Rizzi, F., et al. Chemoprevention of human prostate cancer by oral administration of green tea catechins in volunteers with high-grade prostate intraepithelial neoplasia: a preliminary report from a one-year proof-of-principle study. *Cancer Research.* 66(2):1234–1240, 2006.

23. Klaunig, J. E. Chemopreventive effects of green tea components on hepatic carcinogenesis. *Preventive Medicine.* 21:510–519, 1992.

24. Doucas, H., Garcea, G., Neal, C. P., et al. Chemoprevention of pancreatic can-

cer: a review of the molecular pathways involved, and evidence for the potential for chemoprevention. *Pancreatology.* 6(5):429–439, 2006.

25. Zatonski, W. A., Boyle, P., Przewozniak, K., et al. Cigarette smoking, alcohol, tea, and coffee consumption and pancreas cancer risk. A case-control study from Opole, Poland. *International Journal of Cancer.* 53:601–607, 1993.

Shibata, A., Mack, T. M., Paganini-Hill, A., et al. A prospective study of pancreatic cancer in the elderly. *International Journal of Cancer.* 58:46–49, 1994.

Goto, R., Masuoka, H., Yoshida, K., et al. A case control study of cancer of the pancreas. *Japanese Journal of Cancer Clinics.* 344–350, February 1990.

26. Malaveille, C., Hautefeuille, A., Pignatelli, B., et al. Dietary phenolics as antimutagens and inhibitors of tobacco-related DNA adduction in the urothelium of smokers. *Carcinogenesis.* 17(10):2193–2200, 1996.

Ohno, Y., Aoki, K., Obata, K., et al. Case-control study of urinary bladder cancer in metropolitan Nagoya. *National Cancer Institute Monographs.* 69:229–234, 1985.

27. Busby, J. E., and Kamat, A. M. Chemoprevention for bladder cancer. *Journal of Urology.* 176(5):1914–1920, 2006.

28. Sadzuka, Y., Sugiyama, T., Miyagishima, A., et al. The effects of theanine, as a novel biochemical modulator, on the antitumor activity of adriamycin. *Cancer Letters.* 105:203–209, 1996.

29. The protective effect of "Xin Nao Jian" on the hemogram of cancer patients undergoing radiotherapy and chemotherapy. Jing Fang General Pharmaceutical Company [unpublished].

30. Clinical observation of the treatment of leucocytopenia and thrombocytopenia using Xin Nao Jian Capsule. [unpublished].

CHAPTER 6. TEA'S EFFECT ON CARDIOVASCULAR DISEASE

1. Report of the National Cholesterol Education Program Expert Panel on detection, evaluation, and treatment of high blood cholesterol in adults. *Archives of Internal Medicine.* 148:36–69, 1988.

2. Halliwell, B. Oxidation of low-density lipoproteins. Questions of initiation, propagation, and the effect of antioxidants. *American Journal of Clinical Nutrition.* 61:670–677, 1995.

Regnstrom, J., et al. Susceptibility to low-density lipoprotein oxidation and coronary atherosclerosis in man. *Lancet,* 339:1183–1186, 1992.

3. Frankel, E., Kanner, J., German, J., et al. Inhibition of oxidation of human low-density lipoprotein by phenolic substances in red wine. *Lancet.* 341:454–457, 1993.

4. Muramatsu, K., Fukuyo, M., Hara, Y. Effect of green tea catechins on plasma cholesterol level in cholesterol-fed rats. *Journal of Nutritional Science & Vitaminology.* 32:613–622, 1986.

Fukuo, Y., Kobayashi, Y., Nakazawa, Y., et al. Serum lipoprotein metabolism in long-term users of high cholesterol diet (3 egg yolks and green tea). *Domyaku Koka.* 10:981–988, 1982.

5. Hertog, M. G., Kromhout, D., Aravanis, C., et al. Flavonoid intake and long-term risk of coronary heart disease and cancer in the Seven Countries Study. *Archives of Internal Medicine.* 155:381–386, 1995.

6. Hertog, M. G., Feskens, E. J., Hollman, P. C., et al. Dietary antioxidant flavonoids and risk of coronary heart disease. The Zutphen Elderly Study. *Lancet.* 342:1007–1011, 1993.

7. Kuriyama, S., Shimazu, T., Ohmori, K., et al. Green tea consumption and mortality due to cardiovascular disease, cancer, and all causes in Japan: the Ohsaki study. *Journal of the American Medical Association.* 296(10):1255–1265, 2006.

8. Peters, U., Poole, C., and Arab, L. Does tea affect cardiovascular disease? A meta-analysis. *American Journal of Epidemiology.* 154:495–503, 2001.

9. Sesso, H. D., Gaziano, J. M., Liu, S., et al. Flavonoid intake and the risk of cardiovascular disease in women. *American Journal of Clinical Nutrition.* 77(6):1400–1408, 2003.

10. Imai, K., and Nakachi, K. Cross sectional study of effects of drinking green tea on cardiovascular and liver diseases. *British Medical Journal.* 18, 310:693–696, March 1995.

11. Davies, M. J., Judd, J. T., Baer, D. J., et al. Black tea consumption reduces total and LDL cholesterol in mildly hypercholesterolemic adults. *Journal of Nutrition.* 133(10):3298S–3302S, 2003.

12. Kono, S., Shinchi, K., Ikeda, N., et al. Green tea consumption and serum lipid profiles. A cross-sectional study in Northern Kyushu, Japan. *Preventive Medicine.* 21:526–531, 1992.

13. Stensvold, I., Tverdal, A., Solvoll, K., et al. Tea consumption. Relationship to cholesterol, blood pressure, and coronary and total mortality. *Preventive Medicine.* 21:546–553, 1992.

14. Green, M. S., and Harari, G. Association of serum lipoproteins and health-related habits with coffee and tea consumption in free-living subjects examined in the Israeli CORDIS study. *Preventive Medicine.* 21:532–545, 1992.

15. Miura, S., Watanabe, J., Tomita, T., et al. The inhibitory effects of tea polyphenols (flavan-3-ol derivatives) on $Cu2+$ mediated oxidative modification of low density lipoprotein. *Biological & Pharmaceutical Bulletin.* 17(12):1567–1572, 1994.

16. Yokozawa, T., and Dong, E. Influence of green tea and its three major components upon low-density lipoprotein oxidation. *Experimental and Toxicologic Pathology.* 49:329–335, 1997.

17. Ikeda, I., Imasato, Y., Sasaki, E., et al. Tea catechins decrease micellar solubility and intestinal absorption of cholesterol in rats. *Biochimia et Biophysica Acta.* 1127:141–146, 1992.

18. Hakim, I. A., Alsaif, M. A., Alduwaihy, M., et al. Tea consumption and the prevalence of coronary heart disease in Saudi adults: results from a Saudi national study. *Preventive Medicine.* 36(1):64–70, 2003.

19. Geleijnse, J. M., Launer, L. J., Van der Kuip, D. A., et al. Inverse association of tea and flavonoid intakes with incident myocardial infarction: the Rotterdam Study. *American Journal of Clinical Nutrition.* 75(5):880–886, 2002.

20. Geleijnse, J. M., Launer, L. J., Hofman, A., et al. Tea flavonoids may protect against atherosclerosis: the Rotterdam Study. *Archives of Internal Medicine.* 159:2170–2174, 1999.

21. Sesso, H. D., Gaziano, J. M., Buring, J. E., Hennekens, C. H. Coffee and tea intake and the risk of myocardial infarction. *American Journal of Epidemiology.* 149:162–167, 1999.

22. Mukamal, K. J., Maclure, M., Muller, J. E., Sherwood, J. B., and Mittleman, M. A. Tea consumption and mortality after acute myocardial infarction. *Circulation.* 105:2476, 2002.

23. Huxley, R. R., and Neil, H. A. The relation between dietary flavonol intake and coronary heart disease mortality: a meta-analysis of prospective cohort studies. *European Journal of Clinical Nutrition.* 57:904–908, 2003.

24. Ali, M., and Afzal, M. A potent inhibitor of thrombin stimulated platelet thromboxane formation from unprocessed tea. *Prostaglandins Leukotrienes & Medicine.* 27(1):9–13, 1987.
25. Ali, M., Afzal, M., Gubler, C. J., et al. A potent thromboxane formation inhibitor in green tea leaves. *Prostaglandins Leukotrienes & Essential Fatty Acids.* 40(4):281–283, 1990.
26. Lou, F. Q., Zhang, M. F., Zhang, X. G., et al. A study on tea-pigment in prevention of atherosclerosis. *Chinese Medical Journal.* 102(8):579–583, 1989.
27. Sagesaka-Mitane, Y., Miwa, M., and Okada, S. Platelet aggregation inhibitors in hot water extract of green tea. *Chemical & Pharmaceutical Bulletin.* 38(3):790–793, 1990.
28. Duffy, S. J., Keaney, J. F. Jr., Holbrook, M., et al. Short- and long-term black tea consumption reverses endothelial dysfunction in patients with coronary artery disease. *Circulation.* 104:151–156, 2001.
29. Hodgson, J. M., Puddey, I. B., Burke, V., et al. Regular ingestion of black tea improves brachial artery vasodilator function. *Clinical Science.* 102(2):195–201, 2002.
30. Sims, E. Mechanisms of hypertension in the syndromes of obesity. *International Journal of Obesity.* 5(suppl 1):9, 1981.
31. Stensvold, I., Tverdal, A., Solvoll, K., et al. Tea consumption. Relationship to cholesterol, blood pressure, and coronary and total mortality. *Preventive Medicine* 21:546–553, 1992.
    Henry, J. P., and Stephens-Larson, P. Reduction of chronic psychosocial hypertension in mice by decaffeinated tea. *Hypertension.* 6(3):437–444, 1984.
    Abe, Y., Umemura, S., Sugimoto, K., et al. Effect of green tea rich hi gamma-aminobutyric acid on blood pressure of Dahl salt-sensitive rats. *American Journal of Hypertension.* 8:74–79, 1995.
32. Fitzpatrick, D. F., Hirschfield, S. L, Ricci, T., et al. Endothelium-dependent vasorelaxation caused by various plant extracts. *Journal of Cardiovascular Pharmacology.* 26:90–95, 1995.
33. Keli, S. O., Hertog, M. G., Feskens, E. J., et al. Dietary flavonoids, antioxidant vitamins, and incidence of stroke. *Archives of Internal Medicine.* 154:637–642, 1996.
34. Sato, Y., Nakatsuka, H., Watanabe, T., et al. Possible contribution of green tea drinking habits to the prevention of stroke. *Tohoku Journal of Experimental Medicine.* 157(4):337–343, 1989.
35. Clinical observation of treating cerebral infarction using tea polyphenol (Xin Nao Jian) capsule. Beijing Ji Shui Tan Hospital. [unpublished].

CHAPTER 7. LONGEVI-TEA

1. Sadakata, S., Fukao, A., and Hisamichi, S. Mortality among female practitioners of Chanoyu (Japanese "Tea-ceremony"). *Tohoku Journal of Experimental Medicine.* 166:475–477, 1992.
2. Uchida, S., Ozaki, M., Akashi, T., et al. Effects of (-)-epigallocatechin-3-O-gallate (green tea tannin) on the life span of stroke-prone spontaneously hypertensive rats. *Clinical and Experimental Pharmacology and Physiology.* 22:S302–S303, 1995.
3. Harman, D. Aging and disease. Extending the functional life span. *Annals of the New York Academy of Sciences.* 786:321–336, 1996.
4. Goldbohm, R. A., Hertog, M. G., Brants, H. A., et al. Consumption of black tea and cancer risk. A prospective cohort study. *Journal of the National Cancer Institute.* 88(2):93–100, 1996.

Mukhtar, H. Consumption of black tea and cancer risk. A prospective cohort study. *Journal of the National Cancer Institute.* 88(11):768, 1996.

5. Zheng, W., Doyle, T. J., Kushi, L. H., et al. Tea consumption and cancer incidence in a prospective cohort study of postmenopausal women. *American Journal of Epidemiology.* 144(2):175–182, 1996.

6. Kono, S., Shinchi, K., Ikeda, N., et al. Green tea consumption and serum lipid profiles. A cross-sectional study in Northern Kyushu, Japan. *Preventive Medicine.* 21:526–531, 1992.

7. Green, M. S., and Harari, G. Association of serum lipoproteins and health-related habits with coffee and tea consumption in free-living subjects examined in the Israeli CORDIS study. *Preventive Medicine.* 21:532–545, 1992.

8. Hertog, M. G., Feskens, E. J., Hallman, P. C., et al. Dietary antioxidant flavonoids and risk of coronary heart disease. The Zutphen Elderly Study. *Lancet.* 342:1007–1011, 1993.

 Stensvold, I., Tverdal, A., Solvoll, K., et al. Tea consumption. Relationship to cholesterol, blood pressure, and coronary and total mortality. *Preventive Medicine.* 21:546–553, 1992.

9. Schwarz, B., Bischof, H., and Kunze, M. Coffee, tea, and lifestyle. *Preventive Medicine.* 23:377–384, 1994.

10. Stapleton, P. D., Shah, S., Hamilton-Miller, J. M., et al. Anti-*Staphylococcus aureus* activity and oxacillin resistance modulating capacity of 3-O-acyl-catechins. *International Journal of Antimicrobial Agents.* 24(4):374–380, 2004.

 Sudano Roccaro, A., Blanco, A. R., Giuliano, F., et al. Epigallocatechin-gallate enhances the activity of tetracycline in staphylococci by inhibiting its efflux from bacterial cells. Antimicrobial *Agents and Chemotherapy.* 48(6):1968–1973, 2004.

 Pillai, S. P., Pillai, C. A., Shankel, D. M., and Mitscher, L. A. The ability of certain antimutagenic agents to prevent development of antibiotic resistance. *Mutatation Research.* 496(1–2):61–73, 2001.

11. Pike, J., and Chandra, R. K. Effect of vitamin and trace element supplementation on immune indices in healthy elderly. *International Journal for Vitamin & Nutrition Research.* 65:117–120, 1995.

 Meydani, S. N., Wu, D., Santos, M. S., et al. Antioxidants and immune response in aged persons. Overview of present evidence. *American Journal of Clinical Nutrition.* 62:1462S–1476S, 1995.

12. Hu, Z., Toda, M., Okubo, S., et al. Mitogenic activity of (–)-epigallocatechin gallate on B-cells and investigation of its structure-function relationship. *International Journal of Immunopharmacology.* 14(8):1399–1407, 1992.

13. Kamath, A. B., Wang, L., Das, H., et al. Antigens in tea-beverage prime human Vgamma 2Vdelta 2 T cells in vitro and in vivo for memory and nonmemory antibacterial cytokine responses. *Proceedings of the National Academy of Sciences USA.* 100(10):6009–6014, 2003.

14. Using tea to fight typhoid. *Tea and Coffee Journal.* 129, July 1923.

 Hamilton-Miller, J. M. T. Antimicrobial properties of tea (Camellia sinensis L.). *Antimicrobial Agents and Chemotherapy.* 39(11):2375–2377, 1995.

 Toda, M., Okubo, S., Ohnishi, R., et al. Antibacterial and bactericidal activities of Japanese green tea. *Japanese Journal of Bacteriology.* 44(4):669–672, 1989.

15. Horiuchi, Y., Toda, M., Okubo, S., et al. Protective activity of tea and catechins against *Bordetella pertussis. Kansenshogaku Zasshi—Journal of the Japanese Association for Infectious Diseases.* 66:599–605, 1992.

 Chosa, H., Toda, M., Okubo, S., et al. Antimicrobial and microbicidal activities of tea and catechins against Mycoplasma. *Kansenshogaku Zasshi—Journal of the Japanese Association for Infectious Diseases.* 66:606–611, 1992.

16. Toda, M., Okubo, S., Ikigai, H., et al. The protective activity of tea catechins against experimental infection of *Vibrio cholerae* O1. *Microbial Immunology.* 36(9):999–1001, 1992.

17. Ikigai, H., Nakae, T., Hara, Y., et al. Bactericidal catechins damage the lipid bilayer. *Biochimia et Biophysica Acta.* 1147:132–136, 1993.

18. Konowalchuk, J., and Speirs, J. I. Antiviral effect of commercial juices and beverages. *Applied and Environmental Microbiology.* 35(6):1219–1220, 1978.

    Mukoyama, A., Ushijima, H., Nishimura, S., et al. Inhibition of rotavirus and enterovirus infections by tea extracts. *Japanese Journal of Medical Science & Biology.* 44:181–186, 1991.

19. Nakayama, M., Suzuki, K., Toda, M., et al. Inhibition of the infectivity of influenza virus by tea polyphenols. *Antiviral Research.* 21:289–299, 1993.

    Nakayama, M., Toda, M., Okubo, S., et al. Inhibition of the infectivity of influenza virus by black tea extract. *Kansenshogaku Zasshi—Journal of the Japanese Association for Infectious Diseases.* 68(7):824–829, 1994.

20. Yamada, H., Takuma, N., Daimon, T., et al. Gargling with tea catechin extracts for the prevention of influenza infection in elderly nursing home residents: a prospective clinical study. *Journal of Alternative and Complementary Medicine.* 12(7):669–672, 2006.

21. Williamson, M. P., McCormick, T. G., Nance, C. L., et al. Epigallocatechin gallate, the main polyphenol in green tea, binds to the T-cell receptor, CD4: Potential for HIV-1 therapy. *The Journal of Allergy and Clinical Immunology.* 118(6):1369–1374, 2006.

22. Nakane, H., and Ono, K. Differential inhibition of HIV-reverse transcriptase and various DNA and RNA polymerases by some catechin derivatives. *Nucleic Acids Symposium Series.* 21:115–116, 1989.

23. Davila, J. C., Lenherr, A., and Acosta, D. Protective effect of flavonoids on drug-induced hepatotoxicity *in vitro*. *Toxicology.* 57(3):267–286, 1989.

    Hayashi, M., Yamazoe, H., Yamaguchi, Y., et al. Effects of green tea extract on galactosamine-induced hepatic injury in rats. *Nippon Ronen Igakkai Zasshi (Japanese Journal of Geriatrics).* 100(5):391–399, 1992.

    Imai, K., and Nakachi, K. Cross sectional study of effects of drinking green tea on cardiovascular and liver diseases. *British Medical Journal.* 310:693–696, 1995.

24. Bu-Abbas, A., Clifford, M. N., Walker, R., et al. Selective induction of rat hepatic CYP1 and CYP4 proteins and of peroxisomal proliferation by green tea. *Carcinogenesis.* 15(11):2575–2579, 1994.

25. Hitokoto, H., Morozumi, S., Wauke, T., et al. Inhibitory effects of condiments and herbal drugs on the growth and toxin production of toxigenic fungi. *Mycopathologia.* 66(3):161–167, 1979.

    Ito, Y., Ohnishi, S., and Fujie, K. Chromosome aberrations induced by aflatoxin B1 in rat bone marrow cells *in vivo* and their suppression by green tea. *Mutation Research.* 222(3):253–261, 1989.

    Prasanna, H. R., Lotlikar, P. D., Hacobian, N., et al. Effect of (+)-catechin, dimethyl sulfoxide, and ethanol on the microsome-mediated metabolism of two hepatocarcinogens, N-nitrosodimethylamine and aflatoxin B1. *IARC Scientific Publications.* 84:175–177, 1987.

26. Chakravarthy, B. K., Gupta, S., and Gode, K. D. Functional beta cell regeneration in the islets of pancreas in alloxan induced diabetic rats by (–)-epicatechin. *Life Sciences.* 31(24):2693–2697, 1982.

Ahmad, F., Khalid, P., Khan, M. M., et al. Insulin like activity in (–)-epicatechin. *Acta Diabetologica Latina.* 26(4):291–300, 1989.

Gomes, A., Vedasiromoni, J. R., Das, M., et al. Anti-hyperglycemic effect of black tea (*Camellia sinensis*) in rat. *Journal of Ethnopharmacology.* 45(3):223–226, 1995.

Virtanen, S. M., Rasanen, L., Aro, A., et al. Is children's or parents' coffee or tea consumption associated with the risk for type 1 diabetes mellitus in children? Childhood Diabetes in Finland Study Group. *European Journal of Clinical Nutrition.* 48(4):279–285, 1994.

27. Iso, H., Date, C., Wakai, K., et al. The relationship between green tea and total caffeine intake and risk for self-reported type 2 diabetes among Japanese adults. *Annals of Internal Medicine.* 144(8):554–562, 2006.

28. Yokozawa, T., Chung, H. Y., He, L. Q., et al. Effectiveness of green tannin on rats with chronic renal failure. *Bioscience, Biotechnology & Biochemistry.* 60(6):1000–1005, 1996.

Yokozawa, T., Oura, H., Hattori, M., et al. Inhibitory effect of tannin in green tea on the proliferation of mesangial cells. *Nephron.* 65:596–600, 1993.

29. Curhan, G. C., Willett, W. C., Speizer, F. E., and Stampfer, M. J. Beverage use and risk of kidney stones in women. *Annals of Internal Medicine.* 128:534–540, 1998.

Curhan, G. C., Willett, W. C., Rimm, E. B., et al. Prospective study of beverage use and the risk of kidney stones. *American Journal of Epidemiology.* 143:240–247, 1996.

30. A clinical report on the treatment of chronic renal insufficiency using tea polyphenol (Xin Nao Jian) capsule with an analysis of 25 cases. Department of Kidney, First People's Hospital of Xiao Shan City, Zhe Jiang Province, China. [unpublished].

31. Observation of the anti-free-radical effect in the treatment of chronic renal insufficiency using tea polyphenol. Long Sai Hospital, Ning Bo, China. [unpublished].

32. Matsuoka, Y., Hasegawa, H., Okuda, S., et al. Ameliorative effects of tea catechins on active oxygen-related nerve cell injuries. *Journal of Pharmacology and Experimental Therapeutics.* 274(2):602–608, 1995.

33. Okello, E. J., Savelev, S. U., and Perry, E. K. In vitro anti-beta-secretase and dual anti-cholinesterase activities of *Camellia sinensis* L. (tea) relevant to treatment of dementia. *Phytotherapy Research.* 18(8):624–627, 2004.

34. Mandel, S., Amit, T., Reznichenko, L., et al. Green tea catechins as brain-permeable, natural iron chelators-antioxidants for the treatment of neurodegenerative disorders. *Molecular Nutrition and Food Research.* 50(2):229–234, 2006.

35. Kimura, K., Ozeki, M., Juneja, L. R., et al. L-Theanine reduces psychological and physiological stress responses. *Biological Psychology.* 74(1):39–45, 2007.

36. Ito, K., Nagato, Y., Aoi, N., et al. Effects of L-theanine on the release of alpha-brain waves in human volunteers. *Nippon Nogeikagaku Kaishi.* 72:153–157, 1998.

37. Ohnishi, S. T., Ohnishi, T., and Ogunmola, G. B. Sickle cell anemia: a potential nutritional approach for a molecular disease. *Nutrition.* 16(5):330–338, 2000.

CHAPTER 8. A "NICE CUP OF TEA" FOR DIGESTION

1. He, Y. H., and Kies, C. Green and black tea consumption by humans. Impact on polyphenol concentrations in feces, blood, and urine. *Plant Foods for Human Nutrition.* 46(3):221–229, 1994.

2. Liu, Z., Li, M., and Zhang, G. An approach to determining the effect on salivary amylase by green tea extract. *Chung Hua Kou Chiang i Hsueh Tsa Chih Chinese Journal of Stomatology.* 30(2):89–91, 1995.

Honda, M., and Hara, Y. Inhibition of rat small intestinal sucrase and alpha-glucosidase activities by tea polyphenols. *Bioscience, Biotechnology & Biochemistry.* 57(1):123–124, 1993.

Kreydiyyeh, S. I., Baydoun, A., and Churukian, Z. M. Tea extract inhibits intestinal absorption of glucose and sodium in rats. *Comprehensive Biochemistry & Physiology.* 108(3):359–365, 1994.

Matsumoto, N., Ishigaki, F., Ishigaki, A., et al. Reduction of blood glucose levels by tea catechins. *Bioscience, Biotechnology & Biochemistry.* 57(4):525–527, 1993.

3. Kubota, K., Sakurai, T., Nakazato, K, et al. Effect of green tea on iron absorption in elderly patients with iron deficiency anemia. *Japanese Journal of Geriatrics.* 27(5):555–558, 1990.

4. Mitamura, T., Kitazono, M., Yoshimura, O., et al. The influence of green tea upon the improvement of iron deficiency anemia with pregnancy treated by sodium ferrous citrate. *Nippon Sanka Fujinka Gakkai Zasshi—Acta Obstetrica et Gynaecologica.* 41(6):688–694, 1989.

5. Fukushima, M., and Tanimura, A. Action and absorption possibility of aluminium in infused green tea, black tea, oolong tea, and instant coffee solution at simulated human gastric juice. *Journal of the Japanese Society for Food Science & Technology—Nippon.* 43(8):939–945, 1996.

Drewitt, P. N., Butterworth, K. R., Springall, C. D., et al. Plasma levels of aluminum after tea ingestion in healthy volunteers. *Food and Chemical Toxicology.* 31(1):19–23, January 1993.

6. Weisburger, J. H., Nagao, M., Wakabayashi, K., et al. Prevention of heterocyclic amine formation by tea and tea polyphenols. *Cancer Letters.* 83:143–147, 1994.

7. Stich, H. F. Teas and tea components as inhibitors of carcinogen formation in model systems and man. *Preventive Medicine.* 21:377–384, 1992.

8. Hara, Y. Effect of tea polyphenols on the intestinal flora. *Up-to-Date Food Processing.* 28 (2), February 1993.

9. Terada, A., Hara, H., Nakajyo, S., et al. Effect of supplements of tea polyphenols on the caecal flora and caecal metabolites of chicks. *Microbial Ecology in Health and Disease.* 6:3–9, 1993.

Hara, H., Orita, N., Hatano, S., et al. Effect of tea polyphenols on fecal flora and fecal metabolic products of pigs. *Journal of Veterinary Medical Science.* 57(1):45–49, 1995.

10. Besra, S. E., Gomes, A., Ganguly, D. K., et al. Antidiarrhoeal activity of hot water extract of black tea (*Camellia sinensis*). *Phytotherapy Research.* 17(4):380–384, 2003.

11. Reimann, H.J., Lorenz, W., Fischer, M., et al. Histamine and acute haemorrhagic lesions in rat gastric mucosa. Prevention of stress ulcer formation by (+)-catechin, an inhibitor of specific histidine decarboxylase in vitro. *Agents & Actions.* 7(1):69–73, 1977.

Maity, S., Vedasiromoni, J. R., and Ganguly, D. K. Anti-ulcer effect of the hot water extract of black tea (*Camellia sinensis*). *Journal of Ethnopharmacology.* 46(3):167–174, 1995.

12. Matsubara, S., Shibata, H., Ishikawa, F., et al. Suppression of *Helicobacter pylori*-induced gastritis by green tea extract in Mongolian gerbils. *Biochemical and Biophysical Research Communications.* 310(3):715–719, 2003.

13. Dryden, G. W., Deaciuc, I., Arteel, G., et al. Clinical implications of oxidative stress and antioxidant therapy. *Current Gastroenterology Reports.* 7(4):308–316, 2005.

14. Hara, Y., and Honda, M. The inhibition of alpha-amylase by tea polyphenols. *Agricultural & Biological Chemistry.* 54(8):1939–1945, 1990.

Notes

15. Rumpler, W., Seale, J., Clevidence, B., et al. Oolong tea increases metabolic rate and fat oxidation in men. *Journal of Nutrition*. 131(11):2848–2852, 2001.

Dulloo, A. G., Duret, C., Rohrer, D., et al. Efficacy of a green tea extract rich in catechin polyphenols and caffeine in increasing 24-h energy expenditure and fat oxidation in humans. *American Journal of Clinical Nutrition*. 70(6):1040–1045, 1999.

16. Chantre, P., and Lairon, D. Recent findings of green tea extract AR25 (Exolise) and its activity for the treatment of obesity. *Phytomedicine*. 9(1):3–8, 2002.

17. Dulloo, A. G., Duret, C., Rohrer, D., et al. Efficacy of a green tea extract rich in catechin polyphenols and caffeine in increasing 24-h energy expenditure and fat oxidation in humans. *American Journal of Clinical Nutrition*. 70(6):1040–1045, 1999.

18. Murase, T., Nagasawa, A., Suzuki, J., et al. Beneficial effects of tea catechins on diet-induced obesity: stimulation of lipid catabolism in the liver. *International Journal of Obesity and Related Metabolic Disorders*. 26(11):1459–1464, 2002.

19. Clinical study of weight loss using Arkogelules green tea. *Rev L'assoc Mon Phyto*. June 1985.

20. Dulloo, A. G., et al. Normal caffeine consumption. Influence on thermogenesis and daily energy expenditure in lean and postobese human volunteers. *American Journal of Clinical Nutrition*. 49:44–50, 1989.

CHAPTER 9. WOMEN, BREW UP A CUP OF TEA . . .

1. Delaisse, J. M., Eeckhout, Y., and Vaes, G. Inhibition of bone resorption in culture by (+)-catechin. *Biochemical Pharmacology*. 35(18):3091–3094, 1986.

Kao, P. C., and P'eng, F. K. How to reduce the risk factors of osteoporosis in Asia. *Chinese Medical Journal*. 55(3):209–213, 1995.

2. Hegarty, V. M., May, H. M., and Khaw, K. T. Tea drinking and bone mineral density in older women. *American Journal of Clinical Nutrition*. 71(4):1003–1007, 2000.

Wu, C. H., Yang, Y. C., Yao, W. J., et al. Epidemiological evidence of increased bone mineral density in habitual tea drinkers. *Archives of Internal Medicine*. 162(9):1001–1006, 2002.

3. Cetta, G., Lenzi, L., Rizzotti, M., et al. *Osteogenesis imperfecta*. Morphological, histochemical and biochemical aspects. Modifications induced by (+)-catechin. *Connective Tissue Research*. 5(1):51–58, 1977.

Stoss, H., Pesch, H. J., and Spranger, J. Treatment of *osteogenesis imperfecta* with (+)-catechin. *Deutsche Medizinische Wochenschrift*. 104(50):1774–1778, 1979.

4. Liao, S., Umekita, Y., Guo, J., et al. Growth inhibition and regression of human prostate and breast tumors in athymic mice by tea epigallocatechin gallate. *Cancer Letters*. 96:239–243, 1995.

Araki, R., Inoue, S., Osborne, M. P., et al. Chemoprevention of mammary preneoplasia. *Annals of the New York Academy of Sciences*. 768:215–222, 1995.

5. Brooks, P. G., Garts, S., Heldfond, A. J., et al. Measuring the effect of caffeine restriction on fibrocystic breast disease. the role of graphic stress telethermetry as an objective monitor of disease. *Journal of Reproductive Medicine*. 26:279–282, 1981.

6. Rossignol, A. M., Zhang J., Chen, Y., et al. Tea and premenstrual syndrome in the People's Republic of China. *American Journal of Public Health*. 79:67–69, 1989.

7. Hirose, M., Hoshiya, T., Akagi, K., et al. Inhibition of mammary gland carcinogenesis by green tea catechins and other natually occurring antioxidants in female Sprague-Dawley rats pretreated with 7,12-dimethylbenz[a]anthracene. *Cancer Letters*. 83:149–156, 1994.

8. Zhang, M., Holman., C. D., Huang, J. P., et al. Green tea and the prevention of breast cancer: a case-control study in southeast China. *Carcinogenesis* (in press), 2007.

9. Seely, D., Mills, E. J., Wu, P., et al. The effects of green tea consumption on incidence of breast cancer and recurrence of breast cancer: a systematic review and meta-analysis. *Intergrative Cancer Therapy.* 4(2):114–155, 2005.

10. Zhang, M., Binns, C. W., and Lee, A. H. Tea consumption and ovarian cancer risk: a case-control study in China. *Cancer Epidemiology, Biomarkers, and Prevention.* 11(8):713–718, 2002.

11. Larsson, S. C., and Wolk, A. Tea consumption and ovarian cancer risk in a population-based cohort. *Archives of Internal Medicine.* 165(22):2683–2686, 2005.

12. Huh, S. W., Bae, S. M., Kim, Y. W., et al. Anticancer effects of (–)-epigallocatechin-3-gallate on ovarian carcinoma cell lines. *Gynecological Oncology.* 94(3):760–768, 2004.

13. Zhang, M., Lee, A. H., Binns, C. W., et al. Green tea consumption enhances survival of epithelial ovarian cancer. *International Journal of Cancer.* 112(3):465–469, 2004.

14. Chan, M. M., Soprano, K. J., Weinstein, K., et al. Epigallocatechin-3-gallate delivers hydrogen peroxide to induce death of ovarian cancer cells and enhances their cisplatin susceptibility. *Journal of Cell Physiology.* 207(2):389–396, 2006.

15. Sugiyama, T., and Sadzuka, Y. Theanine and glutamate transporter inhibitors enhance the antitumor efficacy of chemotherapeutic agents. *Acta Biochimica et Biophysica.* 1653:47–59, 2003.

    Sugiyama, T., and Sadzuka, Y. Theanine, a specific glutamate derivative in green tea, reduces the adverse reactions of doxorubicin by changing the glutathione level. *Cancer Letters.* 212:177–184, 2004.

16. Morley, N., Clifford, T., Salter, L., et al. The green tea polyphenol(–)-epigallocatechin gallate and green tea can protect human cellular DNA from ultraviolet and visible radiation-induced damage. *Photodermatology, Photoimmunology & Photomedicine.* 21:15–22, 2005.

    Katiyar, S. K. Skin photoprotection by green tea: antioxidant and immunomodulatory effects. *Current Drug Targets. Immune, Endocrine and Metabolic Disorders.* 3:234–242, 2003.

17. Zhao, J. F., Zhang, Y. J., Jin, X. H., et al. Green tea protects against psoralen plus ultraviolet A-induced photochemical damage to skin. *The Journal of Investigative Dermatology.* 113(6):1070–1075, 1999.

18. Miyachi, Y. Photoaging from an oxidative standpoint. *Journal of Dermatological Science.* 9:79–86, 1995.

    Gerrish, K., and Gensler, H. Prevention of photocarcinogenesis by dietary vitamin E. *Nutrition and Cancer.* 19:125–133, 1993.

    Makimura, M., Hirasawa, M., Kobayashi, K., et al. Inhibitory effect of tea catechins on collagenase activity. *Journal of Periodontology.* 64(7):630–636, 1993.

19. Ohmori, Y., Ito, M., Kishi, M., et al. Antiallergic constituents from oolong tea stem. *Biological & Pharmaceutical Bulletin.* 18(5):683–686, 1995.

    Chan, M. M., Ho, C., and Huang, H. Effects of three dietary phytochemicals from tea, rosemary, and turmeric on inflammation-induced nitrite production. *Cancer Letters.* 96:23–29, 1995.

    Matsuo, N., Yamada, K., Yamashita, K., et al. Inhibitory effect of tea polyphenols on histamine and leukotriene B-4 release from rat peritoneal exudate cells. *In Vitro Cellular & Developmental Biology.* 32(6):340–344, 1996.

CHAPTER 10. A CUP A DAY KEEPS THE DENTIST AWAY

1. Woodward, M., and Walker, A. R. Sugar consumption and dental caries. Evidence from 90 countries. *British Dental Journal.* 176(8):297–302, 1994.

2. Sato, T., and Niwa, M. Cariostatic mechanisms of fluoride and its effects on human beings. *Japanese Journal of Clinical Medicine.* 54(1):67–72, 1996.

   Chavassieux, P., and Meunier, P. J. Benefits and risks of fluoride supplements. *Archives de Pediatrie.* 2(6):568–572, 1995.

3. Gulati, P., Singh, V., Gupta, M. K., et al. Studies on the leaching of fluoride in tea infusions. *Science of the Total Environment.* 138(1–3):213–221, 1993.

4. Kjellevold Malde, M., Greiner-Simonsen, R., Julshamn, K., et al. Tealeaves may release or absorb fluoride, depending on the fluoride content of water. *The Science of the Total Environment.* 366(2–3):915–917, 2006.

5. Trevisanato, S. I., and Kim, Y. I. Tea and health. *Nutrition Reviews.* 58(1):1–10, 2000.

6. Sarkar, S., Sett, P., Chowdhury, T., et al. Effect of black tea on teeth. *Journal of the Indian Society of Pedodontics and Preventive Dentistry.* 18:139–140, 2000.

7. You, S. Q. Study on feasibility of Chinese green tea polyphenols (CTP) for preventing dental caries. *Chung Hua Kou Chiang i Hsueh Tsa Chih Chinese Journal of Stomatology.* 28(4):197–199, 1993.

   Kitamura, K., Loyola, J. P., and Sobue, S. Inhibitory effects of a hot water extract from Japanese tea on the cell growth of *mutans streptococci. Shoni Shikagaku Zasshi—Japanese Journal of Pedodontics.* 28(3):618–622, 1990.

8. Matsumoto, M., Minami, T., Sasaki, H., et al. Inhibitory effects of oolong tea extract on caries-inducing properties of *mutans streptococci. Caries Research.* 33(6):441–445, 1999.

   Rasheed, A., and Haider, M. Antibacterial activity of *Camellia sinensis* extracts against dental caries. *Archives of Pharmacology Research.* 21(3):348–352, 1998.

9. Otake, S., Makimura, M., Kuroki, T., et al. Anticaries effects of polyphenolic compounds from Japanese green tea. *Caries Research.* 25(6):438–443, 1991.

10. Linke, H. A., and LeGeros, R. Z. Black tea extract and dental caries formation in hamsters. *International Journal of Food Science Nutrition.* 54(1):89–95, 2003.

11. Ooshima, T., Minami, T., Aono, W., et al. Oolong tea polyphenols inhibit experimental dental caries in SPF rats infected with *mutans streptococci. Caries Research.* 27:124–129, 1993.

   Sakanaka, S., Sato, T., Kim, M., et al. Inhibitory effect of green tea polyphenols on glucan synthesis and cellular adherence of cariogenic streptococci. *Agricultural & Biological Chemistry.* 54(11):2925–2929, 1990.

12. Ooshima, T., Minami, T., Aono, W., et al. Reduction of dental plaque deposition in humans by oolong tea extract. *Caries Research.* 28:146–149, 1994.

13. Jones, C., Woods, K., Whittle, G., et al. Sugar, drinks, deprivation and dental caries in 14-year-old children in the north west of England in 1995. *Community Dental Health.* 16(2):68–71, 1999.

14. Yu, H., Oho, T., and Xu, X. Effects of several tea components on acid resistance of human tooth enamel. *Journal of Dentistry.* 23(2):101–105, 1995.

15. Onishi, M., Ozaki, F., Yoshino, F., et al. Experimental evidence of caries preventive activity of nonfluoride component of tea. *Journal of Dental Health.* 31:158–161, 1981.

   Elvin-Lewis, M., and Steelman, R. The anticariogenic effects of tea drinking among Dallas children. *Journal of Dental Research.* 65:198, 1968.

16. Horiba, N., Maekawa, Y., Ito, M., et al. A pilot study of Japanese green tea as a medicament. Antibacterial and bactericidal effects. *Journal of Endodontics.* 17(3):122–124, 1991.

17. Sakanaka, S., Aizawa, M., Kim, M., et al. Inhibitory effects of green tea polyphenols on growth and cellular adherence of an oral bacterium, *Porphyromonas gingivalis. Bioscience, Biotechnology & Biochemistry.* 60(5):745–749, 1996.

Osawa, K., Matsumoto, T., Yasuda, H., et al. The inhibitory effect of plant extracts on the collagenolytic activity and cytotoxicity of human gingival fibroblasts by *Porphyromonas gingivalis* crude enzyme. *Bulletin of Tokyo Dental College.* 32(1):1–7, 1991.

CHAPTER 11. IT'S TEA TIME!

1. Aizaki, T., Osaka, M., Hara, H., et al. Hypokalemia with syncope caused by habitual drinking of oolong tea. *Internal Medicine.* 38(3):252–6, 1999.
2. Taylor, J. R., and Wilt, V. M. Probable antagonism of warfarin by green tea. *Annals of Pharmacotherapy.* 33(4):426–8, 1999.
3. Hyon, S. H. A non-frozen living tissue bank for allotransplantation using green tea polyphenols. *Yonsei Medical Journal.* 45(6):1025–1034, 2004.

Index

Cetta, G., 153
Ch'a Ching (Lu Yu), 28, 32, 33
Chai, 44
Chanoyu (Japanese tea ceremony), 14
Chelating agents, 55
Chemotherapy, 1, 60, 88–91, 121, 157
Chicago, University of, 84
China, 122, 130, 155, 171
  cancer in, 70, 72, 77–80, 89–91, 121, 156
  cardiovascular disease in, 105–6, 110–11
  dementia in, 131
  dental hygiene in, 164–65
  European trade with, 40–43
  green tea varieties from, 177–81
  health claims for tea in, 11
  history of tea use in, 27–35, 40
  influence on Japan of, 36–39
  longevity in, 114
  renal failure in, 130
  tea cultivation in, 4, 5, 45
Cholera, 123
Cholesterol, 2, 12, 94–98, 101–4, 109, 118, 126
  See also HDL-cholesterol; LDL-cholesterol
Chun Mee tea, 177
Cigarettes, *see* Smoking
Cirrhosis, 126
Clostridium, 123
Coffee, 4, 18, 45, 62, 118, 119
Cognitive function, 115, 130–31, 135
Colitis, ulcerative, 146–48
Colon cancer, 13, 14, 63, 64, 78, 80–81, 86, 117, 141
  inflammatory bowel disease and, 147
Coenzyme Q$_{10}$, 48
Congestive heart failure, 107
Coronary artery disease, 93–94, 100, 105–6
Coumadin, 172
Crohn's disease, 137, 146–48
Croton oil, 65
Cruz, Gaspar da, 41

Dayalbagh Educational Institute, 164
Decaffeinated teas, 21, 57, 140, 158, 172, 175–76
Dementia, 131–33

Dental cavities, preventing, 1, 10, 11, 15, 25, 111, 125, 159–68
  fluoride and, 24, 140, 163–64
Desmutagens, 71
Detoxification, 2, 111, 126–27, 135
Diabetes, 10, 108, 115, 128–30
Diarrhea, 15, 122, 142–44
  in Crohn's disease, 146, 147
Diet, 115, 117–19
  Asian, 67, 83, 84, 114
  cancer and, 59, 62–66, 141–42
  cholesterol and, 96, 98–99, 101
  dental cavities and, 162–63, 165
  digestive disorders and, 143–47
  French, 53, 98
  liver disease and, 126
Digestion, 137–50
  disorders of, 15, 142–48
DNA, 50, 51, 60, 64–65, 125
  prevention of damage to, 69–71, 73, 76, 81, 158
Dragon Pearls tea, 178
Dragon Well tea, 178
Duke University, 113
Dutch East India Company, 29, 41

EC, 17, 53, 17, 55, 56, 129
ECG, 17, 55, 56, 158
EDTA, 55
EGC, 17, 55, 56
EGCG, 17, 18, 55–57, 116, 123–25, 131, 158, 172, 173
  cancer and, 65, 71, 77, 80, 82–84, 154, 156, 157
  cardiovascular disease and, 103, 105
  for cavity prevention, 165, 166
  for weight loss, 149
Egypt, history of tea in, 44
Eisai Myoan, 36
Elizabeth I, queen of England, 42
Emerald Petals tea, 178
England, *see* Britain
Environmental toxins, 51, 52, 115, 117, 126
Enzymes, 157, 165
  antioxidant, 52, 58, 70
  digestive, 139, 140, 144, 148
  liver, 72–73, 127
Ephedra, 21
Epicatechin, *see* EC
Epicatechin gallate, *see* ECG

Index

About the Authors

LESTER A. MITSCHER has conjoint academic appointments at the University of Missouri–Kansas City and the Victorian College of Pharmacy, Melbourne, Australia, and publishes actively in the field of herbal medicines. Overall he has published more than 250 research publications and authored or coauthored six technical books on drug discovery and properties. He is a member of the executive committee of the International Organization for Chemistry in Developing Countries and has traveled extensively, lecturing and performing research. He consults in the pharmaceutical industry and for the National Institutes of Health. His research awards include the Smissman Award in Medicinal Chemistry (American Chemical Society), Volweiler Award (American Association for Pharmaceutical Education), the Research Achievement Award in Natural Products Chemistry (American Pharmaceutical Association), the Award in Medicinal Chemistry (Medicinal Chemistry Division, American Chemical Society), and the Career Research Achievement Award (American Society for Pharmacognosy). He is an Elected Fellow of the American Association for the Advancement of Science and a member of the Medicinal Chemistry Hall of Fame of the American Chemical Society.

VICTORIA DOLBY TOEWS, MPH, has been researching and writing about health issues since 1993. She earned a Master in Public Health degree (summa cum laude) from Portland State University, which is a collaborative degree between Oregon Health and Science University, Oregon State University, and Portland State University. She also graduated summa cum laude from Western Oregon University with a Bachelor of Science in Health Education.

As a veteran freelance researcher and writer, she has written or co-authored numerous health and wellness books, including *User's Guide to Healthy Digestion*, *User's Guide to Sexual Satisfaction*, *The Soy Sensation*, *User's Guide to Glucosamine and Chondroitin*, *The Common Cold Cure*, and—of course—the first edition of *The Green Tea Book*. She is also the managing editor for *The Natural Pharmacy, 2nd edition* and *A–Z Guide to Drug-Herb-Vitamin Interactions*.

Her work has been recognized for excellence as a finalist in the 2001 Maggie Awards, which honors editorial excellence in magazines west of the Mississippi River, and she was awarded the Oregon Laurels Scholarship, 1995–1998. She has written hundreds of magazine articles about achieving wellness through natural medicine and dietary supplements.

Victoria, her husband, Jeff, and their children live in the Pacific Northwest, where they enjoy cycling, hiking, and cross-country skiing.